OXFORD MEDICAL PUBLICATIONS

GARROD'S INBORN FACTORS IN DISEASE

OXFORD MONOGRAPHS ON MEDICAL GENETICS

General Editors:
ARNO G. MOTULSKY   MARTIN BOBROW
PETER S. HARPER   CHARLES SCRIVER

Former Editors:
J. A. FRASER ROBERTS   C. O. CARTER

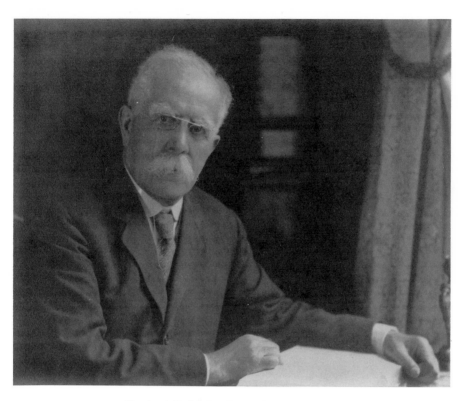

Sir Archibald E. Garrod 1858–1936
*(Original Photograph taken in 1934,
courtesy of Simon Garrod.)*

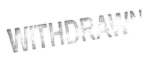

OXFORD MONOGRAPHS ON MEDICAL GENETICS · 16

GARROD'S INBORN FACTORS IN DISEASE

Including an annotated facsimile reprint of

THE INBORN FACTORS IN DISEASE

by

ARCHIBALD E. GARROD

CHARLES R. SCRIVER
Professor of Biology, Human Genetics, and Paediatrics,
McGill University, Montréal, Québec, Canada

and

BARTON CHILDS
Emeritus Professor of Paediatrics,
The John Hopkins University School of Medicine,
Baltimore, Maryland, USA

OXFORD   NEW YORK   TORONTO   TOKYO
OXFORD UNIVERSITY PRESS
1989

Oxford University Press, Walton Street, Oxford OX2 6DP

Oxford New York Toronto
Delhi Bombay Calcutta Madras Karachi
Petaling Jaya Singapore Hong Kong Tokyo
Nairobi Dar es Salaam Cape Town
Melbourne Auckland

and associated companies in
Berlin Ibadan

Oxford is a trade mark of Oxford University Press

Published in the United States
by Oxford University Press, New York

British Library Cataloguing in Publication Data
Scriver, Charles R. (Charles Robert), 1930–
Garrod's inborn factors in disease.
1. Man. Diseases. Genetic factors
I. Title II. Childs, Barton
616'.042
ISBN 0–19–261574–2

Library of Congress Cataloging in Publication Data
Garrod, Archibald E. (Archibald Edward), Sir, 1857–1936.
[Inborn factors in disease]
Garrod's inborn factors in disease : including an annotated
facsimile reprint of The inborn factors of disease by Archibald E.
Garrod/[edited, with new material by] Charles R. Scriver and
Barton Childs.
(Oxford monographs on medical genetics; 16)
(Oxford medical publications)
A companion vol. to: Garrod's inborn errors of metabolism.
Includes bibliographies.
1. Disease susceptibility. 2. Medical genetics. I. Scriver,
Charles R. II. Childs, Barton. III. Garrod, Archibald E.
(Archibald Edward), Sir, 1857–1939. Inborn errors of metabolism.
IV. Title. V. Title: Inborn factors in disease. VI. Series.
VII. Series: Oxford monographs on medical genetics; no. 16.
[DNLM: 1. Disease Susceptibility—familial & genetic.
QZ 50 G2431 1931a] RG151.G3 1989 616'.042—dc19 88–29102
ISBN 0–19–261574–2

Typeset by Latimer Trend & Company Ltd, Plymouth
Printed and bound in Great Britain by
Biddles Ltd, Guildford and King's Lynn

FOREWORD

JOSHUA LEDERBERG
President
The Rockefeller University, New York

The reissue of Archibald Garrod's prescient work is most timely. We are at the very brink of unlimited access to molecular polymorphisms in DNA as the key to the ultimate analysis of human individuality, in health and in disease.

No one could be better qualified than Barton Childs and Charles Scriver to undertake the task of this new edition in view of their individual contributions to human genetic science, their evangelism on the necessity of genetic understanding in medical and in humanistic education, and of their finely tuned appreciation of the significance of Garrod's previsions in the history of ideas.

Inborn factors in disease should be read as a companion to Garrod's earlier and broader work, *Inborn errors of metabolism* (1909), which has been made available to contemporary readers through Professor Harry Harris's 1963 edition. As indicated by the titles, *Metabolism* recites the specific biochemical–genetic syndromes—alcaptonuria having been the prototype—that established the concept of biochemical individuality. *Disease* is more particularly addressed to practitioners and philosophers of medicine. It gathers the later but more diffuse and fragmentary evidence to relate individuality to 'diathesis', that is to genetically based predispositions to a broad range of disease. With particular foresight, Garrod included infectious disease and other syndromes unlikely to have a simple genetic aetiology, and where complex interactions with environment were inevitable.

Garrod's theory of the gene is tantalizing. In his earlier works, metabolic deviations were 'sports'; it is difficult to divine exactly what he believed to be the scope and function of the normal gene(s). Many biologists were asserting that Mendelian genes only influenced the variability found within a species, the group

[v]

within which hybridization could test the hypothesis. The relationship of chromosomal genes to the totality of influence on development by the cytoplasm was still argued. In *Disease*, p. 147, he does however assert:

Seeing that all factors in the constitution of the future man are represented in the chromosomes of the germinal cells from which he shall spring, it can hardly be supposed that such diverse potentialities as are afforded in structures so minute, and so little different from each other as are the germinal cells of creatures of different species, can have other than a molecular representation.

This is not yet the direct one to one mapping of genes to enzymes later insisted on by Beadle and Tatum. It is a powerful assertion of the primacy of the chromosome. We do not know the evidence on which he relied; and we cannot even be sure of the subtlety of his reasoning—whether he had considered and rejected the Plasmon concept, viz. that the cytoplasm still transmitted the basic architecture common to larger taxons than the species (Sapp 1987). Garrod was, in small detail, in error: we might quibble that not quite all the genetic constitution is in the chromosomes; some tiny proportion is in the mitochondrial genome. The irony is that these exceptions prove the rule—the primacy of DNA whether in the nuclear chromosomes or in extranuclear plasmids.

The intensity of neglect of Garrod's thought by his contemporaries has, perhaps, been exaggerated. Nevertheless, it is obvious that it has received far more attention since the 1940s in the wake of (1) the modern era of experimental biochemical genetics opened up by Beadle and Tatum's work with Neurospora in 1941, and (2) the new wave of human genetic study epitomized by Neel's (1949) and Pauling and Itano's (Itano *et al.* 1949) work on sickle cell disease. Beadle (1958) records his surprise at how many of his and Tatum's ideas had been anticipated by Garrod—and it is not that they can have been totally unaware of them (Lederberg 1989), though most likely they knew of them second-hand through Haldane's 1937 review which they cite in their 1941 paper. Haldane's remarks may help illuminate some of the constraints on the impact of Garrod's

ideas: '[his] pioneer work on congenital human metabolic abnormalities such as alcaptonuria and cystinuria had a very considerable influence both on biochemistry and genetics. But alcaptonuric men are not available by the dozen for research work. . . . '
That is, one must await more tractable experimental tools, such as
Neurospora was soon to furnish, to enable a laboratory imple-
mentation of Garrod's way of thinking. Haldane was already
quite exceptional in his gift for an amenability to speculation.
Few scientists have that patience. In fact, through unhappily
evolutionary drama, dozens of men with sickle cell disease and
trait were all too readily available—one but had to know to look
there.

By the 1930s Garrod's *Metabolism* had been cited in a handful
of textbooks—one or two in genetics, a few more in biochemistry. The most influential of these were probably Bodansky
(1934) and R. J. Williams (1931); the latter was followed by a
number of books advocating attention to biochemical individuality (see Williams 1956). *Disease* was hardly cited at all: a brief
notice in the *New England Journal of Medicine* (May 9, 1931) recites:
'The whole subject is still extremely complicated and although
Garrod's analysis is helpful, little is added to our knowledge. The
book is pleasantly written and is a scholarly contribution'.

In view of the modest shrift given genetics teaching in many
medical schools, and the muddiness of many nature–nurture
debates even to this day, we should not be too smug about the
inattentiveness to Garrod almost 60 years ago. Today, even more
than ever, many more ideas are afloat than any mortal can
reasonably attend to; in that competition for attention, many
wonderful foresights will inevitably be neglected. They may be
saved from oblivion by noisy assertiveness, by perseverant
accumulation of compelling data, or by unpredictable fashions of
popularity. Accidents of circumstance or of personality assure
that many eventual winners are today's 'premature' insights. The
most vulnerable to deterrence are those that require a spanning of
disciplines beyond customary teaching. Today, the sheer population density of science may militate against the neglect afforded a
Mendel or a Garrod; it is difficult to find more contemporary

FOREWORD

examples. On the other hand, scientific and medical education becomes every day more specialized; the 'project system' gate-keeping of academic careers places heavy burdens on the would-be interdisciplinarian, and weightier burdens still on the speculative thinker.

As certain as I am of new diamonds in our dust, few are likely to be of the lustre exhibited in *Inborn factors of disease*.

REFERENCES

Beadle, G. W. (1958). Genes and chemical reactions in Neurospora. *Les Prix Nobel* 147–59.
Beadle, G. W. and Tatum, E. L. (1941). Genetic control of biochemical reactions in Neurospora. *Proceedings of the National Academy of Sciences USA* **27**, 499–506.
Haldane, J. B. S. (1937). The biochemistry of the individual. In *Perspectives in biochemistry* (ed. J. Needham and D. E. Green, pp. 1–10. Cambridge University Press, Cambridge. This article was cited by Beadle and Tatum in 1941.
Lederberg, J. (1989). *Edward Lawrie Tatum (December 14, 1909–November 7, 1975)*. Biographical Memoirs, National Academy of Sciences, Vol. 59. National Academy of Sciences, Washington DC.
Neel, J. V. (1949). The inheritance of sickle cell anemia. *Science* **110**, 64–6.
Pauling, L., Itano, H. A., Singer, S. J. and Wells, I. C. (1949). Sickle cell anemia: a molecular disease. *Science* **110**, 543–8.
Sapp, J. (1987). *Beyond the gene. Cytoplasmic inheritance and the struggle for authority in genetics*. Oxford University Press, Oxford.
Williams, R. J. (1931). *An introduction to biochemistry*. Van Nostrand, New York.
Williams, R. J. (1956). *Biochemical individuality: the basis for the genotype concept*. Wiley, New York.

PREFACE: SETTING THE SCENE

Our theme is inherited susceptibility or resistance to disease in humans. It concerns a body of reliable knowledge that will serve as a basis for action, can lead to correct prediction, and is relevant to choices of action that matter. We use here John Ziman's definition of reliable knowledge (Ziman 1979).

Our theme is actually Garrod's own, stated by him at length, albeit in a different context, in the book republished here. It seems, with hindsight, to be an obvious book, one that would have had an easy emergence and success. It was otherwise, in the event.

'I assented palely . . . I don't see how we can very well avoid doing it . . . It ought not to cost more than £100 (to publish) and might even sell a few copies.' Thus an internal memorandum, dated 1 November 1927, recorded Garrod's intention to write 'a work of science, not a work of practical medicine' which the author wished to offer as 'a parting gift' to the Delegates of the Oxford University Press. (In those days medical books were not published by the part of the press overseen by the delegates.) The occasion for the offer was the Huxley Lecture on the subject of *diathesis* which Garrod would deliver at the Charing Cross Hospital on 27 November 1927. The memorandum continues: 'I understand (diathesis) means "constitutional liability to disease" . . . a subject long neglected owing to interest in germs and like attacking forces'. In due course, *The inborn factors in disease* was published. The date was 1931.

With the hindsight of half a century and more, one must admire the publisher. He was dealing with one of the most respected physicians of the day and he perceived the novelty of Dr Garrod's theme, but he knew his market! Physicians were not likely to be greatly interested in 'a work of science', and even if they were, they would probably have trouble with the great man's theme and variation on inherited predisposition owing to their overriding concern with 'germs and like attacking forces'

[ix]

PREFACE

which were still important causes of disease in their patients.

Although the original invitation from the Press to ourselves in the mid 1980s was to reprint, for a second time with a new commentary, Garrod's equally remarkable but better known first book, *Inborn errors of metabolism*, we suggested that the Press republish *The inborn factors in disease*. We preferred *Inborn factors* because we believe there is a developing context in which diathesis makes sense today. Genes are now in every person's vocabulary; the Watson–Crick model of DNA, the mechanisms of inheritance, and the genotype–phenotype paradigm are all central to our view of biology; and at the root of all disease is biology.

The barrier that the practising physician encounters when tackling Garrod's *Inborn factors* is the concept of diathesis; yet genetic predisposition—for that is what is meant by diathesis— should not be strange. As our adviser at the Press said when we discussed the project, everyone can see that the new grandchild has the family nose, eyes, whatever;* why then is the family nose familiar yet the family disease is not? Even on this point, Garrod was perceptive: he recognized that few of us know 'our' diseases even though we could discover them by diligent enquiry (p. 63, *Inborn factors*).

* Thomas Hardy also said it, in a poem:

> *Heredity*
> I am the family face;
> Flesh perishes, I live on,
> Projecting trait and trace
> Through time to times anon,
> And leaping from place to place
> Over Oblivion.
>
> The years-heired feature that can
> In curve and voice and eye
> Despise the human span
> Of durance—that is I;
> The eternal thing in man,
> That heeds no call to die.

In *Moments of vision* (1917)

[x]

PREFACE

The reader of *The inborn factors in disease* will see that Garrod's view of diathesis is a logical extension of his enveloping idea about chemical individuality. One could say that *Inborn factors* bears a relationship to *Inborn errors* corresponding to that between multifactorial and monogenic diseases. And just as Mendelian phenotypes are yielding to analysis by molecular genetic methods, so will the multifactorial diseases wherever genetic determinants are an important component of their cause. In the context of molecular genetics a reprint of *Inborn errors* is timely.

Access to methods that are diagnostic of cause is only one facet of the context that makes *Inborn factors* cogent. Another is relevance. As the consequences of 'germs and the like attacking forces' are diminished by public health measures and better treatments, the development of corresponding measures for so-called 'genetic' diseases becomes an abiding concern. Garrod does not discuss prevention in *Inborn factors* perhaps because it was fruitless to do so (moreover he could not know how), but that is no longer the case. Garrod did not anticipate the events of today, but he did describe an hypothesis with examples that are now both valid and useful. Science, as in history, through the deposit of knowldge affects the present. The present affects our perception of the past. Medicine has its own past and in its science—Garrod's designated context for *Inborn factors*—the past has affected the present. It is time to appreciate what Garrod wrote and to understand why the book that 'failed' then need not have that fate now.

The records of the Oxford University Press mention that 1250 copies of the original book were printed; the stock was exhausted by June 1938. Where are those 1000 odd copies now? We know very few persons who have actually read *Inborn factors* and only a few others apparently know of it. We located through computerized records of library accessions less than a dozen copies of the book in North America. To be deprived any longer of Garrod's graceful prose and his perceptive thinking in *Inborn factors* is a lapse needing correction. We hope there will be many readers of this reprint and that the Press will be gratified by sales.

Our version of *Inborn factors* has five sections. First, this Preface

[xi]

PREFACE

to set the scene. Then, a Prologue in which we describe Garrod's aims for the book and the limitations of the knowledge within which he presented his interesting ideas. Garrod's book itself follows. Then comes an Epilogue in which we show how chemical individuality is the reality claimed by Garrod and how widely it accounts for diathesis or predisposition to disease. Finally, for those who wish to learn more about this interesting man there are two Bibliographies: one of his own papers, many of which still make absorbing reading; the other of articles about Garrod's career and his ideas which continue to influence us. Some readers may prefer to read Garrod's book first and then go to other sections. To place the book immediately after the Preface represented an alternative plan, but we decided upon the present arrangement assuming that many readers might prefer some introduction to Garrod and his times.

This book did not spring fully armed from our brows. It reflects discussions between ourselves and with colleagues, teachers, and students over many years. We owe a special debt to Joshua Lederberg who contributed substantially to the text describing Garrod's view of genes; and to Simon Garrod, great grand nephew of Archibald E. Garrod and Reader in Psychology at Glasgow University, who further illuminated our view of Sir Archibald and provided the previously unpublished photograph for the frontispiece. We thank the staff of the Press for their patience and many helpful suggestions, and Lynne Prevost, Emily Pasterfield, and Huguette Rizziéro for converting pages of squiggles and scratches into neat typescript. Lastly we thank our Universities, granting agencies, and our families for the gifts of time to discover Garrod.

Charles R. Scriver
McGill University
Montreal

Barton Childs
John Hopkins University
Baltimore

CONTENTS

[xiii]

CONTENTS

PROLOGUE: GARROD IN CONTEXT

Owing, as I believe, to their chemical individuality different human beings differ widely in their liability to individual maladies, and to some extent in the signs and symptoms which they exhibit. [Garrod 1926]

Sir Archibald E. Garrod, KCMG, DM, LLD, FRCP, FRS was educated to be a physician. He also trained himself in physiological chemistry to be a scientist. His medical experience brought him face to face with patients and his scientific enquiries led him to find explanations for some of their diseases. His excellent training combined with a capacity to make novel observations permitted him to develop the robust concept of chemical individuality which he applied to the interpretation of disease throughout a long and exceptionally productive career (Goldstein 1986). His colleague and informal mentor, Sir Frederick Gowland Hopkins, often referred to as the father of biochemistry, said of Garrod in a brief memoir for the Royal Society, 'With all his predilection for experimental science Garrod remained first and foremost a clinician with a deep sense of the dignity and importance of that calling. When speaking, as he often did, of the help that Medicine receives from Science he was always concerned to emphasize the view that this is but a repayment of the debt that Science has owed to Medicine' (Hopkins 1938). In this Prologue we place Garrod in context showing him as the physician–scientist who, because of his time and its lack of the knowledge essential to translate his concept into practice, was forced to write a book that was 'a work of science, not a work of practical medicine'.

Garrod was called upon may times to deliver named lectures and to speak to an important occasion. The theme of the lectures and of his scientific papers published after the turn of the century was consistent: chemical individuality was a major determinant of health and disease in human kind. This view and the evidence for it emerged in his studies of alcaptonuria and blossomed in the

[1]

Croonian Lectures and two editions of *Inborn errors of metabolism.** The mature flowering of chemical individuality as a concept came in the Huxley lecture on diathesis, and in the book that followed it—*The inborn factors in disease*. One can readily trace the growth of the idea and the evidence from which it came by comparing the first book with the second. Garrod placed the concept of diathesis or genetic predisposition, as he expounded it in *Inborn factors*, in the domain of science, and he did not see his second book as a work of practical medicine. History shows that *Inborn factors* was not a success in its day either as a scientific book or as a medical treatise because the necessary evidence was lacking to vindicate the scientific underpinning of the book and the methods required to gain the evidence would come only half a century later. But the evidence has now made Garrod's ideas relevant to medicine. The patients, all of whom are the children of parents and who in their turn may be parents of children, are the beneficiaries.

The epigraph to the Prologue is taken from an address given by Garrod to the entering class of medical students at Westminster Hospital, on 1 October 1926. He had been giving important lectures for almost two decades and, although the students would probably not have known it, the Westminster Hospital Lecture rings changes on the familiar Garrod peal; perhaps the Faculty recognized this. Garrod's lecture ends with this thought: 'for the clinical as for the laboratory worker, and especially for both working in cooperation, there is abundant scope for original investigation—that highest product of the scientific spirit'. Garrod was inviting every physician whether formative or mature, to be a student of variation, to the benefit of the patient. His own experiences as a physician had led him to know there were ample opportunities to make original observations that concern the cause of disease. It was true then and it is still true.

Throughout Garrod's writings, there is a conceptual tension. He was both a physician interested in the familiar medical signs and symptoms of disease and a scientist who had discovered unusual causes which could underlie the common manifestations

* Citations of Garrod's writing refer to the Bibliography of his writings.

of disease, and he wrote accordingly. In his role as a scientist he used the idiosyncratic to explain the common in medical practice; as a physician, he was able to find novelty in common things. The dual role was probably as difficult to play then as it is now. It is as apparent now as when Professor Harris edited the 1963 reprint of *Inborn errors*, that genetics has continued to advance rapidly. 'When a subject is rapidly advancing', Harris said, 'it is interesting and often instructive to look back and reread some of the early contributors, where ideas which now seem commonplace were first formulated'. In the late 1980s, one cannot help but believe that molecular genetics provides a tangible link between Garrod's view of disease, which he developed in *Inborn factors*, and its modern application to the theory and practice of medicine. The *Inborn factors in disease* may have been the culmination of Garrod's own intellectual voyage which began before *Inborn errors of metabolism* but we see it as the beginning of a collective journey in medicine for which this reprint is merely a signpost.

GARROD: THE PERCEPTIVE PHYSICIAN—SCIENTIST

The primary question in the practice of medicine always was, is, and will be: 'Why does *this* patient have *this* disease, *now*?' The question is more commonly put in another form: 'What *disease* does this patient have and how do I *treat* it?' Garrod linked Mendelian concepts with an appreciation that inherited traits, expressed in the form of chemical individuality, could be diseases or at least predispositions to them and thereby he answered the first question very well. From his scientific vantage-point he was the ideal physician because he recognized that the patient with the disease is something different from the disease the patient has. Garrod's message has been rather cryptic for physicians, and perhaps overinterpreted by geneticists. Accordingly, we thought it was useful to discriminate between what Garrod actually said, the apparent limits of his knowledge about inherited cause of disease, and the light shed on medical practice by what he said and did. But before doing so we should state the case for Garrod as an influential physician in his own times, something rather different than the prophet of biochemical-genetics-before-his-time so admired by many of us.

What the world thinks of a man is revealed in his obituaries. How his contemporaries remembered Sir Archibald E. Garrod is apparent in notices which appeared in several journals (*Lancet* 1936; *British Medical Journal* 1936; Hopkins 1936*a, b*, 1938; *St. Bartholomew's Hospital Reports* 1936).* The fact that four were in medical journals (including Hopkins 1936*a*) indicates that Garrod's contributions to medicine were considered important by his peers;† on the other hand, none of the medical notices gives the impression that Garrod's major contribution to medicine was his concept of human chemical individuality and of how that singularity can constitute an inherited predisposition to disease.

The medical notices, in particular, imply that Garrod was more scientist than physician. The *Lancet* (1936) writer records that 'patients, as he himself said, did not really interest him and a solution to their disease did not really appeal'; further on, that 'he wondered also, how he had come to be a practising physician'; and again, 'In a patient he saw one symptom only, one abnormality, and on this he would concentrate, thinking about it, reading about it, and experimenting with it, all else ignored'. Whether these are the qualities we admire in a physician or not, Garrod's peers were obviously admiring of these qualities because he was appointed successor, in 1920, to Sir William Osler as Regius Professor of Physic at the University of Oxford. In the *Saint Bartholomew's Hospital Reports* one learns that: '(Medical) problems were always discussed (by him) from a scientific standpoint, and the traditional views were not accepted without careful thought'. Garrod's habit was 'to delve into the causes of the disease and symptoms' and it is appropriate that he was joint editor of *The Quarterly Journal of Medicine* from 1907 to 1929. It is

---

* *St. Bartholomew's Hospital Reports* (1936) contains a complete bibliography of Garrod's scientific writings (republished here).

† The three obituaries contributed by Sir Frederick Gowland Hopkins (1936*a, b*, 1938) indicate the respect of one great scientist for another.

[4]

the imperceptive reader who is not aware that cause and mechanism of disease rather than manifestations were Garrod's abiding interest in medicine.

Garrod showed his inclination to delve into the events underlying manifestations of disease in his famous study of alcaptonuria. According to the author of the *St. Bartholomew's Hospital Report*:

A little while before 1898 (Garrod's) interest in urinary pigments brought him in touch with a case of alkaptonuria and this was responsible for his great work for medicine. At that time nearly all diseases were thought to be due to infective agents and alkaptonuria was supposed to be caused by an organism in the intestines which disturbed the metabolism of tyrosin, and was thus responsible for the excretion of homogentisic acid. One afternoon while walking home from the hospital thinking about these problems, it suddenly occurred to him that alkaptonuria might be due to a chemical error on the part of the body which might be present throughout life.

Garrod's insight had its origin in observations made on one of his alcaptonuria patients. The patient was a newborn infant in whom the appearance of homogentisic aciduria was followed from birth; the chemical abnormality was clearly evident 52 hours after birth (Garrod 1901). Garrod surmised that the chemical finding was congenital—not acquired. He then observed that parental consanguinity was more common than usual among parents of children with alcaptonuria (Garrod 1901). In the clue hidden in the first-cousin marriages, lore has it that Garrod quickly recognized the Mendelian nature of alcaptonuria. This is unlikely because, in 1901, Garrod was apparently unaware of the relation between Mendel's work and his own findings (Bearn and Miller 1979). But Bateson was sufficiently aware and he interpreted Garrod's cases as evidence for inheritance of a recessive character (Bateson 1901–02). There was correspondence between Bateson and Garrod on the issue of consanguinity but, according to Bearn and Miller (1979), it is unclear who initiated it and whether the precedent for thinking about chemical individuality in Mendelian terms is Garrod's or Bateson's. However, it is clear that, in due course, in thinking about a *manifestation* (alcapto-nuria), Garrod had identified a *pathogenetic process* (a biochemical error) and had deduced that its *cause* (or, as he saw it, the consequence) was inherited.

From this significant beginning Garrod went on to build his general case for chemical individuality in man which he presented first in the Croonian Lectures (1908) and then in *The inborn errors of metabolism* (1909). And on that foundation, he built an edifice which he would call 'the higher medicine' in the Linacre Lecture at Cambridge in 1923. On that occasion, he attributed to the advances in bacteriology and protozoology revelations about causes of disease, new methods to combat it, and the advent of preventive medicine and aseptic surgery. He observed that the new medicine had also benefited from advances in endocrinology and nutrition, and in a telling phrase he proposed that 'pathology is anatomy and physiology gone wrong' (Garrod 1923).

His view of pathology is significant. Progress in biochemistry had helped him, in his own work, to see pathological processes in terms of molecules while, as a student, he had been taught to think of pathology in terms of cells. In one of those mysterious leaps of insight, Garrod developed the theme that proteins possess the required complexity to be vehicles of biological individuality. In his role as the Linacre lecturer he tells us that different species have haemoglobins with different properties of crystallization; he knew that the property of individuality resided in the globin and not in the haeme moiety. Garrod goes so far as to say there would be 'special proteins for every species and indeed for every individual in a species'. (This idea precedes the evidence for protein polymorphisms and molecular heterozy-gosity by many years!) He went on to encourage the view that 'bodily form and chemical structure go hand in hand'.

How the transmission of phenotype might occur was also within Garrod's sphere of interest and he spoke about it, again in the Linacre lecture.

It seems to me that the strongest argument that can be adduced in support of the hypothesis that bodily form depends on chemical structure is based on the fact that the germinal cells of different animals, which resemble each other so closely in structure, and even the chromosomes of their nuclei, obviously include factors which determine both the forms and metabolic peculiarities of the organisms which originate from them.

As he proceeds in the lecture he offers this idea:

If it may be granted that the individual members of a species vary from the normal of the species in chemical structure and chemical behaviour, it is obvious that such variations or *mutations* are capable of being perpetuated by *natural selection*; and not a few biologists of the present day assign to chemical structure and function a most important share in the *evolution of species*. [Our italics.]

It is inappropriate to attribute the novelty of these ideas solely to Garrod. They were current among the biologists of this day (*vide infra*). The novelty lies in his adept application of them to medicine. In the same lecture, after dealing with inborn errors of metabolism, he goes on to say:

Very few individuals exhibit such striking deviations from normal metabolism as porphyrinurics and cystinurics show, but I suspect strongly that minimal deviations which escape notice are almost universal. How else can be explained the part played by heredity in disease? There are some diseases which are handed down from generation to generation ... which tend to develop in later childhood and early adult life ... It is difficult to escape the conclusion that although these maladies are not congenital, their underlying causes are inborn peculiarities.

Garrod ends the Linacre lecture with a balanced argument. First, he cites examples of external influences which can be counted among the causes of disease—bacteria, protozoa, chemical poisons, trauma, and radiant energy, in other words those hazards related to unwanted exposure to materials and energy in the environment (the 'germs and like attacking forces' referred to by his editor). Garrod then proceeds to this idea:

But in addition to all these, there need to be taken into account factors inherent in our patients. Thus, we are led back to something very like

[7]

the doctrine of diatheses which was so much in vogue in the days of our grandfathers, but has fallen into disrepute, and finds little or no place in the medical teaching of today. In the 'New English Dictionary' diathesis is defined as 'a permanent (hereditary or acquired) condition of the body which renders it liable to certain diseases, or affections; a constitutional predisposition or tendency'. In this limited sense I, for my part, am compelled to admit the truth of the doctrine. *In short diathesis is only another name for chemical individuality.* [Our italics.]

'Glimpses of the higher medicine' (The Linacre lecture), from which the preceding passages are taken, was delivered on 5 May 1923. On 24 November 1927 Garrod delivered the Huxley Lecture, titled 'On diathesis', at Charing Cross Hospital. Further thinking from this fruitful point of view ultimately yielded *The inborn factors in disease* in 1931. It was Garrod's last major publication.

GARROD IN CONTEXT

All this has a very modern sound; indeed, the Oxford University Press is republishing *The inborn factors in disease* because the book represents so precisely what is emerging as modern thought about disease. But in that modern sound lie the enigmas that clothe Garrod's contributions. First, why were his ideas not embraced by his contemporaries, or even his successors, and, second, what exactly did he mean by the things he wrote and said, as opposed to what, given our up-to-date knowledge, he might *seem* to us to mean?

Garrod's non-acceptance

Stent (1972) has suggested that a discovery will fail to be accepted if ' . . . its implications cannot be connected by a series of simple logical steps to canonical, or generally accepted, knowledge'. The idea of inborn errors could, and did, make such a connection with the biochemists of Garrod's time, but in genetics and medicine it did not (Fruton 1972; Olby 1974). The idea of chemical individuality was apparently accepted by no one.

[8]

GARROD IN CONTEXT

Biochemistry

The notion that an enzyme deficiency might cause a variation or a disease, while entirely novel, did not lie completely counter to the conventional wisdom, or at least it was possible to take in; it did no violence to the principles of metabolism in pathways, for example. Nor was Garrod alien to the biochemists. At a meeting of the Historical Section of the Royal Society of Medicine in 1931, Gowland Hopkins described Garrod as one of the two fathers of biochemistry (the other was Liebig) (Brit. Med. J. 1932a). Perhaps the position is best described in Table 1 which shows references to Garrod in 20 textbooks of biochemistry available in the Johns Hopkins Medical Library and published between 1901 and 1945. Apparently, it took some time for the message to disseminate; most of the citations were to the second edition of *Inborn errors of metabolism* published in 1923. The table also suggests that the flow was limited; about two-thirds failed to mention him or his work. This limitation extends also to the citations themselves; Garrod's writing was nearly always quoted, not in support of basic principles of biochemistry, but as illustrations of biochemical attributes of disease. All references were to one or more of the inborn errors; only one author listed

TABLE 1. References to Garrod in biochemistry textbooks published before 1945.

Year published	Reference to Garrod		Total
	No	Yes	
1901–10	1	1	2
1911–20		1	1
1921–30	4	1	5
1931–40	6	4	10
1941–45	2		2
Total	13	7	20

[9]

the *Lancet* paper of 1902 and *no one* mentioned chemical individuality despite the prominent display of the idea in so many of Garrod's publications from 1902 on. No doubt some of this failure is due to parochial reading habits; biochemists may not have read the *Lancet* or the *British Medical Journal*, and such titles as *Inborn errors of metabolism* or *Inborn factors in disease* might easily have failed to attract their notice.

Genetics

Garrod concluded that alcaptonuria and other inborn errors were inherited according to Mendelain modes, so, within a few years of the rediscovery of Mendelism, there were several hereditary human conditions, all called inborn errors and all presumed to be enzyme deficiencies. This was an auspicious beginning, but one that seems to have died at birth.

The field of genetics was at that time so rudimentary that these ideas should have had as good a chance for acceptance as any, but a vital connection was lacking—a link between the inferred protein (enzyme) deficiency and something that could be called a gene. That is, before Garrod's ideas could be accepted by geneticists, the physical basis of genetics—mutation, recombination, linkage, sex linkage, and so on—had to be established and all that, of course, lay in the future. Although the chromosomal basis was clarified as early as 1902, the elaboration of the facts of inheritance went on over a period of two decades or so, mainly through the study of drosophila by Morgan and his colleagues, and it was not until the 1920s and 30s that geneticists were ready to focus on how the genes act. That is, by the 1930s it was possible to approach the problem of gene action experimentally and based upon a solid ground of genetics, whereas Garrod's conclusions, outlined in his 1909 book, had to be inferential. We know that his ideas were never mentioned by the Morgan school, and Moore has suggested that, even if Morgan knew of the inborn errors, he might have ignored them because the hypothesis they posed could not be tested by breeding experiment (Moore 1986). There were other pioneer studies in biochemical genetics; anthocyanin pigments accounting for flower colours (Haldane 1937; Scott-Moncrieff 1981–83) and melanins for the coat colours of animals (Wright 1941) were subjected to genetic analysis, but these efforts were not much better received than Garrod's. So, in addition to the lack of a purely genetic context in which to fit his ideas, there was the lack of biochemical understanding on the part of the geneticists, a deficiency not remedied much before the late 1930s (Haldane 1937) and early 1940s (Wright 1941). Perhaps that is why Garrod's part in what came to be called physiological genetics was so late in being acknowledged.

There is a second reason. Mendelian inheritance was not quickly accepted. At first it did not fit in with contemporary ideas which were dominated by Galton's theory of ancestrian heredity (Froggatt and Nevin 1971). The Galtonians, who studied only continuous variation, concluded that, although what was transmitted was particulate, inheritance was blending so that no segregation was possible. Furthermore, they could not accept that mutation, which was a rare event anyway, could account for evolution which they believed must occur in infinitesimally small steps. To Bateson, the essence of Mendelism was mutation and segregation, and he became a forceful, even belligerent, advocate of evolution by saltation. There ensued a bitter, acrimonious debate between the ancestrians and the Mendelists which could not be resolved until Fisher published his 1918 paper in which he demonstrated that both continuous and discontinuous variation were explainable by the segregation of independent genes (Froggatt and Nevins 1971). Garrod's position in this contention is unknown, but he was a Mendelist and, in proposing chemical individuality, he was suggesting that everyone differed from everyone else in a variety of ways and not necessarily in continuous distributions. And it is not clear that Garrod's cause was furthered by the violence of Bateson's advocacy. Nor was it helped by the presence–absence explanation of gene action (Olby 1974). Bateson proposed that dominance could be explained by the presence of a factor (later, gene), the absence of which accounted for recessive effects. Multiple alleleism and pairing at meiosis could not accommodate the presence–absence hypothesis, so it was given up by everyone but Bateson, who, in his dogged way, persisted in proclaiming it until he died (Bateson 1926). Again, we do not know how Garrod's views on presence –absence evolved, but the idea of the inborn errors may have been tainted by association (Olby 1974).

Medicine

It is an amusing paradox that, despite his salience as Regius Professor of Physic at Oxford and the evident respect accorded him by everyone in his profession, Garrod's ideas were almost completely overlooked by physicians. They were overlooked because they could not be perceived; in medical circles the inborn errors were considered altogether in the context of disease, and from that point of view a few rare, more or less harmless peculiarities expressed in the urine or skin just did not loom as issues of consuming importance. It is easy to understand how the sublety of inborn errors and chemical individuality could escape the notice of contemporary physicians taken up with overwhelming and devastating disease.

Preoccupation with life-threatening, often untreatable, disease is evident in the edition of *Modern medicine* (Osler and McCrae 1925) and *Osler's principles and practice of medicine* (McCrae 1935), published contemporaneously with *Inborn factors*. Two-fifths of the pages of these textbooks are devoted to infections for which there was then no specific treatment. This is in contrast to the 10th edition of *Harrison's principles of internal medicine* (Petersdorf *et al.* 1983) in which only one-tenth of the space is given to infections and a nearly equal amount is accorded to disorders Garrod would have recognized as inborn errors of metabolism. Further, the idea of host susceptibility and resistance to infections, to which Garrod devoted a chapter in *Inborn factors*, and which is certainly taken seriously in the 1980s must, in the early 1930s, have evoked only an incredulous response from his readers. Everyone knew then that infections were due to virulent micro-organisms that attacked, and sometimes killed, human

[12]

beings. It was sufficient to know that and not necessary to enquire further about host factors.

In *Inborn factors*, Garrod added several diseases to his list of inborn errors; he included gout, Gaucher's disease, haemophilia, and porphyrinuria. Of these and the original four, all but albinism and porphyrinuria are mentioned in Osler, sometimes with the designation 'inborn error, (Garrod)', so it cannot be said that the diseases were unknown. Rather, it was the idea and its implications that could not be taken in.

A second reason for the lack of grasp of these ideas is that they could not be tested. Doctors, then as now, are practical and are mainly interested in what can be applied to the daily round of patient care. There is little to feed other than the mind in most of Garrod's writing, but even the intellectual stimulus was in some ways abortive because the ideas existed only as hypotheses that could not be tested. Medes described tyrosinosis in 1932 and Fölling published his observations of phenylpyruvic oligophrenia (phenylketonuria) in 1934. But it was not until the 1950s, when it became possible to separate and to measure proteins, amino acids, sugars, and other substances and to assay enzyme activity, that the discovery of new inborn errors began to climb along an exponential curve to reach our present state of knowledge. A comparison of the 1909 edition of *Inborn errors* with the fifth edition of a modern classic reference, *The metabolic basis of inherited disease* (Stanbury *et al.* 1983) shows the difference (Table 2).

The development of our understanding of chemical individuality did not follow the acceptance of the idea of the inborn error. It took a different path beginning with the discovery of the blood group substances and their genetic control, then taking impetus from Pauling's demonstration of the molecular variation of haemoglobins and from the electrophoretic separation of serum proteins and enzymes, and culminating in the current proliferation of variations in the DNA. But, in contrast to the inborn errors which came eventually to fit so neatly into the medical view of homeostasis, it was the genetic analysis that made sense of what turned out to be a truly extensive variation among

TABLE 2. Evidence of modern acceptance and extension of the idea of inborn errors

	Garrod (1909) *Inborn errors of metabolism,* first edition	Stanbury *et al.* (1983) *The metabolic basis of* *inherited disease,* fifth edition
Date of publication	1909	1983
No. inborn errors	4	200
Weight	300 g	3060 g
Contributors	1	137
Chapters	6	91
Pages	168	2048
Surface area (sq in)	9300	143 000
Words	40 000	1 300 000
References	248	20 369
Refs./chapter	41	250
Index, pages	11	34
Index, items	600	6900
Cost (1985 US dollars)	$2.50	$95.00
Cost/kg of book (US dollars)	$9.00	$31.10

proteins. This formulation we owe to Harris (1980b) for man and Lewontin (1985) for drosophila. Despite the apparent lack of relationship between the organisms they studied, both groups concluded that about 30 per cent of loci specifying soluble enzymes showed two or more alleles, the least frequent of which occurred at a frequency of 1 per cent. This meant that each individual should be heterozygous for such alleles at about 7 per cent of loci. It was agreed that, because the methods fail to detect all differences, this might be a considerable underestimate. Others have since shown the variability to be both less for structural proteins and greater for DNA sequences.

So during the past 30 years investigators, drawn from all three of the disciplines (biochemistry, genetics, and medicine) into which Garrod's hypotheses might have fitted when they were first proposed, have collaborated to attain a degree of confirmation of his ideas that even he might not have imagined to be possible.

[14]

But it is not solely in the vindication of his ideas that we are so comfortable with Garrod today. He is astonishingly modern in other ways—ways that must have helped to make him incomprehensible to his contemporaries.

First, the idea of chemical individuality, once accepted, bends one's thought in certain directions, foreclosing others. One such consequence is the desire to explain the whole by reference to its parts, and Garrod was emphatically an early reductionist. He saw variation of all kinds as due to chemical events, whether enzyme action or antibody production, and even physical differences were laid to such account. This is expressly the modern aim in which phenotype variations are traced to differences in the structure of DNA. Reductionist ideas were not much in fashion in Garrod's time. Many scientists, perhaps mainly physiologists, thought there were principles of life that reduction to chemical reactions could not reveal. One such physiologist, J. S. Haldane (the father of J. B. S. Haldane) was a powerful advocate of such a view; 'Those who aim at physico-chemical explanations of life are simply running their heads at a stone wall and can only expect sore heads as a consequence' (Fruton 1972, pp. 491–2). But among those who differed with Haldane and who perceived the need to explain physiology in terms of biochemical processes was Garrod's colleague and friend, Gowland Hopkins (Fruton 1972, p. 492). We might know a good deal more about Garrod had someone been able to record his conversations with Hopkins.

Second, the idea of chemical individuality was (and still is) more compatible with the thinking of evolutionists than with that of physicians. Physicians then (and to too great a degree still) thought in terms of classes: there were the healthy and the sick; among the sick were those classed as tuberculous, others with duodenal ulcer or with haemophilia, and so on. What were important were the differences between the classes, not within. Such thinking has been called typological by Mayr, and it is to be contrasted with population thinking in which variation within classes is as significant as that between (Mayr 1980). Mayr says, 'Unless one adopts population thinking and considers every individual as representing a uniquely different genotype, natural

[15]

selection does not make sense' (Mayr 1980, p. 29). Again and again, Garrod asserted that what distinguishes human beings one from another is chemical individuality and in *Inborn factors* (in the section on evolution and disease pp. 52–60), he made clear his acceptance of natural selection (p. 53). This is more remarkable than it might seem to us today because in his time many thought otherwise. Bateson, for example, rejected natural selection, believing that evolution proceeded by mutation alone, and there were others, evolutionists among them, who accepted the inheritance of acquired characters as an additional route to evolution (Mayr 1980). So Garrod was a thorough-going population thinker in an age of typology.

A third consequence of the idea of chemical individuality is its strong support for the historical, or physiological, concept of disease. Since antiquity disease has been observed from two points of view (Temkin 1963; King 1982). In one version, called ontological, diseases have entity; they are real things, they can be identified by their characteristics, they attack a previously healthy person, and each victim is seen to be representative of the class. In the alternative version, called historical, physiological, or nominalist, disease is envisioned as a quantitative variation in an individual, the extent of which is determined by that person's specific response to experience. If every person is different (e.g. chemical individuality) then the disease expression will vary accordingly. Garrod nowhere acknowledges these contrasting views, but chemical individuality is incompatible with the ontological concept and wholly at one with the alternative. Today, evidences of chemical individuality, taking the form of genetic and other risk factors, are accumulating rapidly, and disease is increasingly acknowledged to be a consequence of incongruence between a genetically influenced homeostasis and the conditions of living. Today, it is entirely ' . . . justifiable to claim that what our fathers called diathesis is only another name for chemical individuality' (*Inborn factors*, p. 122).

[16]

GARROD IN CONTEXT

WHAT WAS IN GARROD'S MIND?

In giving body to the idea of chemical individuality, Garrod described differences in proteins between species and suggested that such variation should exist between human beings. Further, he said that chemical individuality should be a reflection of molecular differences that characterize the chromosomes. All this sounds remarkably like what we accept today, but we lack any direct insight into his mind. His words could have meant one thing to him when he uttered them and something else to us who are tempted to freight them with contemporary significance. So, since modern technology has yet to perfect a means of communication with our forebears, we can only examine their words the more closely and try to interpret what they *could* have meant, given the information available and the intellectual context of the time.

Olby suggested that, in the study of the history of ideas, it is too easy to accord the earliest outline of a principle the same status as a later and fuller account based on information obtained in the meantime (Olby 1974, p. 435). This error he calls 'precursor disease' and Garrod's writing offers ample opportunity to make such slips. For example, Garrod has been given credit by Beadle for being the first to propose a direct relationship between a gene and an enzyme; 'In this roundabout way, first in drosophila, then in neurospora, we had rediscovered what Garrod had seen so clearly, so many years before' (Beadle 1959). But, in fact, Garrod could not have made any such proposal in 1909 and there is no evidence in *Inborn factors* or in the lectures given in the 1920s that he came to that conclusion later on. Indeed, his attitude to genetics is ambiguous; we do not know how much he knew or understood of developments after about 1910. For example, he seldom, if ever, used the word gene, preferring 'factor', which by 1931 had been long discarded. Certainly by that time the physical basis of inheritance was well worked out; indeed Morgan's first book (written with Sturtevant, Muller, and Bridges) was published in 1915, and by the end of the 1920s there was abundant

[17]

information defining genes, their position in chromosomes, their relationships to each other, and their segregation in gametes. But Garrod mentions drosophila only once in *Inborn factors* (p. 42), and that in relation to the recurrence of mutations, and no reference is given. Instead he refers to Mendel, Galton, and Bateson. On page 61 we find, 'some of the chief difficulties which, until recent times, surrounded the study of inheritance have now been overcome, thanks to the work of Francis Galton and Gregor Mendel, and those who have carried on so assiduously the researches they initiated'. We simply do not know which 'assiduous' investigators he meant. Also on page 61, while deploring a lack of space to discuss ' ... modern views on heredity ... ', he says, 'it will be necessary ... to assume that the reader has at least some acquaintance with the Mendelian theory and the views of Galton ...'; no mention of the views of Morgan. Nor is our confidence bolstered by his reference on page 67 to Bateson's presence–absence theory, even though it is to say that it presents some difficulty. Furthermore, there are no references to Wheldale's or Scott-Moncrieff's work on the genetics of antho-cyanin pigments or to Wright's study of genetic variation in coat colours in mammals. For example, in a book called *The anthocyanin pigments of plants* published in 1916, Wheldale said, ' ... we have now, on one hand, satisfactory methods for the isolation, analyses and determination of the constitutional formulae of these pig-ments. On the other hand, we have the Mendelian methods for determining the laws of their inheritance. By a combination of these two methods we are in reasonable distance of being able to express some of the phenomena of inheritance in terms of chemical composition and structure' (cited in Scott-Moncrieff 1981–3). And in 1917 Wright published a paper called 'Color inheritance in mammals', in which appears the sentence, ' ... color variations of nearly every kind have been shown to be due genetically to variations in the enzyme element of the reaction that produces pigment'. It is curious that not one of these three originators of biochemical genetics cited the other. It is a further example of what Merton calls 'multiples', in which two or more people make the same discovery, each in ignorance of the other

(Merton 1961). But by 1931, when *Inborn factors* was published, geneticists were beginning to focus on physiological genetics, which is to say, gene action (Wright 1941).

So, if Garrod did not envision the genetic apparatus as it had been described by the drosophilists he could not have given the inborn errors the precision of one gene–one enzyme. What he did do was to make the connection between one hereditary protein variation and one bit of chemical individuality, and if he didn't add the third element, the gene, well, how much is one man supposed to do? The advantage Beadle and Tatum had in their quest was a detailed knowledge of the *genetics* of drosophila and neurospora (Beadle 1945; ibid. 1959). Indeed, they started with drosophila because it was the best characterized organism from the genetic vantage. Had they begun with Garrod's one enzyme (protein)—one bit of chemical individuality in mind, the job relating a single gene to a single enzyme might have been a good deal easier. It seems that no one investigator read the other's literature; if Garrod did not know of the plant and animal pigment work, neither did others know of his. (The way science is organized today makes such neglect virtually impossible.)

What are we to make of Garrod's frequent reference to molecular groupings ' . . . which confer upon us our individualities, and which went to the making of the chromosomes from which we sprang'. In the germ cells these 'molecular groupings' were 'proteins, nucleotides and lecithin', while in the somatic cells the proteins are singled out. 'It is the extreme complexity of the molecules of the proteins . . . that makes it possible to imagine how chemical individuality can exist' (*Inborn factors*, p. 44). He goes on to say that the possibilities for combinations of amino acids are akin to the numbers with which astronomers deal, and then, 'It cannot be doubted that natural selection works through chemical as well as structural modifications, nor that the features in which an organism differs from type are foreshadowed in the molecular complexes in the chromosomes'. (There are echoes here of the Linacre Lecture.) It sounds as if he conceived of some sort of affinity between chromosomal molecules and chemical individuality, and that the relationship was mediated by proteins.

[19]

This idea was not wholly new, having been suggested earlier (Troland 1917), but it is more nearly guesswork, however inspired, than the idea of the inborn errors. The latter could fit handily enough into contemporary biochemistry, the former could not. It could not, because the issues of peptide linkage and amino acid sequence were unsettled until the 1940s and neither was it known to Garrod that tertiary structure was determined by amino acid sequence (Fruton 1972, pp. 148–79). Thus, whatever his idea was, it was not of any sort of colinear relationship between molecules in the germ cells and proteins, or that the structure of proteins could be the determinant of how they function. What he did know is that species were characterized by the composition of their proteins, and he suggested that such differences ought also to define individuals. A brilliant insight, but one that was neither testable nor, apparently, appealing to investigators of his time.

Some final questions remain. What did Garrod expect of his book? What did he hope medical practitioners would take from it and how might they use the information? These questions are answered at the end of the Prologue where he suggests that some understanding of diathesis or innate predisposition must help the doctor to ' . . . recognize the qualities and individual needs of his patients' (*Inborn factors*, p. 23). And the last paragraph in this section reads, 'Wittingly or unwittingly, the practitioner of medicine is constantly engaged in the study of constitutions and predispositions, and of reactions to environment. He must, throughout his active life, be a student of the inborn as well as of the external factors of disease' (p. 24). To which today we should all say, 'Of course'. Whether we are such students, whether the Westminster Hospital students were, is another matter.

But how was the book received? In the United Kingdom, the book was reviewed in the *British Medical Journal* (1932*b*) and *Lancet* (1932), and in the United States, by the *New England Journal of Medicine* (1932) and the *Journal of the American Medical Association* (1931). Both of the American reviews were short, 10 and 14 lines respectively, and both were devoid of any inkling of the book's message or purpose. The *Lancet* review was somewhat better, but undid its good work by concluding with the following: ' ... to those to whom the dull and laborious task of accumulating human genetical data does not appeal, we commend Draper's method of exploring the association between particular diseases and the different types of bodily configuration'. Garrod devoted about one page of *Inborn factors* to Draper's work; it was in no way central to his ideas and argument. The review in the *British Medical Journal* was about one and one-third pages long and recited most of the principles presented in the book. Of the four reviews, it was the only one that could possibly have aroused the interest of a potential reader or caused anyone to buy the book. All four commented on the graceful writing.

We know nothing of how Garrod himself felt about this failure of the reviewers to grasp his ideas. Perhaps his own sense of fulfilment was not wrapped up in acceptance of the ideas by medical colleagues. He was, after all, Regius Professor, gave all the most prestige-laden lectures in his homeland, served on its most exalted committees, and was a consultant of last resort. Also, he did know that some biochemist friends had some idea of what was going on in his mind. And he may have resigned himself to his fate, knowing from first-hand experience that rare hereditary conditions could not command the attention of practitioners who daily confronted overwhelming disease without the means to combat it, and that inborn predispositions to disease were of only abstract interest to those who lacked any means to prevent their onset.

What has happened since Garrod's death? Between 1955 and 1984 the citation index lists 1013 references to Garrod's papers and books, a respectable showing indeed. Of these references about one-half were to the Croonian lectures, about one-fifth to the two volumes of *Inborn errors*, and one-tenth to the 1902 *Lancet* paper. In addition, about 19 per cent of the citations referred to his many other papers. But there were only 15 references to *Inborn factors*, a little over 1 per cent of the total. Eleven of the papers making these 15 citations were conveniently available and of the 11, 10 were taken up with Garrod's conception of gout as an

[21]

inborn error of metabolism. Only one made much of his themes of chemical individuality, susceptibility, and diathesis. That limited view of Garrod's ideas could change now that we are on the threshold of a detailed description of the human genome. Such knowledge should greatly enhance our understanding of the causes of disease and, with it, our knowledge of pathogenesis will increase too. The idea of chemical individuality has been given an empirical basis, and we are about to use the information for purposes which Garrod would approve. That is why the Oxford University Press is making *Inborn factors* available to the modern reader.

THE INBORN FACTORS
IN DISEASE

THE INBORN FACTORS
IN DISEASE

AN ESSAY

BY

ARCHIBALD E. GARROD, K.C.M.G.

D.M., LL.D., F.R.C.P., F.R.S.

Consulting Physician to St. Bartholomew's
Hospital, and to the Hospital for Sick Children;
sometime Regius Professor of Medicine in
the University of Oxford

OXFORD

AT THE CLARENDON PRESS

1931

[27]

OXFORD UNIVERSITY PRESS
AMEN HOUSE, E.C. 4
LONDON EDINBURGH GLASGOW
LEIPZIG NEW YORK TORONTO
MELBOURNE CAPETOWN BOMBAY
CALCUTTA MADRAS SHANGHAI
HUMPHREY MILFORD
PUBLISHER TO THE
UNIVERSITY

PRINTED IN GREAT BRITAIN

[28]

PREFACE

THIS essay had its origin in the Huxley Lecture on 'Diathesis' delivered by its author at the Charing Cross Hospital in 1927.

In it the bearings of more recent scientific advances upon the problems of disease are discussed more fully than was possible in a single lecture.

Its pages reflect the outlook of a student of medicine of fifty years' standing who began his medical studies shortly before the discovery of the tubercle bacillus, and has witnessed the advances of, and the profound changes in, medicine and surgery during the most fruitful half-century in their history.

The author takes this opportunity to express his sincere gratitude to all those who have helped him in various ways, and especially to Sir Frederick Andrewes and Professor F. R. Fraser for their valued criticism and advice.

December 1930.

CONTENTS

[31]

Prologue

THE DOCTRINES OF DIATHESIS

Dupes d'un mot, les médecins ont cru pendant longtemps, et la plupart croient encore avoir donné la clef de ces phénomènes aussitôt qu'ils ont dit: Ce sont des diathèses, et cette croyance empêche d'en chercher une autre explication.—L. F. ROCHE. 1831.

FAR back, in the early days of medical knowledge, it was recognized that some individuals are more, and others less liable to this or that disease; and it was known at least as early as the commencement of the Christian era, that diseases may be handed down from parents to children.

Towards the end of the eighteenth century, at a time when clinical medicine was beginning to be set upon a firmer basis than it had had for centuries previously; not only by increased study of morbid anatomy, but also by the introduction of new methods for the detection of local lesions, and especially auscultation and percussion, there was also a great awakening of interest in less tangible matters, the morbid predispositions and the so-called temperaments.

At that time, and indeed through the greater part of the nineteenth century, it was in the French Schools of Medicine that such matters were most actively discussed, and much of the discussion centred around the word 'diathesis'.[1]

[1] For an admirable history of the Doctrines of Diatheses, *see* André Leri, *Progrès Méd.*, 1912, xl. 141 et seq.

No little interest attaches to the history of this phase of medical doctrine, although it appears to us to-day that much of the pursuit of the diatheses was carried out in a fog, and led the pursuers along tangled ways. At any rate some account of the stages of the pursuit is highly desirable, if not essential, as an introduction to any discussion of the inborn factors in disease, as these appear when examined in the light of more recent scientific advances.

Widely different meanings have been attached to the word diathesis,*at different times, in different countries and medical schools, and even by individual members of the same school. These differences are largely re-sponsible for the disfavour into which the term has fallen; they are so fundamental that they deprive the name diathesis of all practical utility; and reluctant as one must needs feel to abandon a time-honoured desig-nation, this particular one has become so damaged by conflicting uses that its employment, in any modern sense, is calculated to lead to fresh confusion. That being so, it seems better to lay it aside.

It may be recalled that the original meaning of διάθεσις, was an arrangement of objects in space, their disposition, and hence *a* disposition. In more recent usage, the meaning attached to the word has been a dis-position, or predisposition, to a particular malady or group of maladies. It is in this sense that it has been employed by the great majority of English writers and teachers.

* *diathesis* For whatever reason(s), the word diathesis has been 'laid aside'. But into the vacuum has rushed the expression 'risk factors'. Today's genetic risk factors are the descendants of the nineteenth century's diatheses.

[34]

Thus, in some manuscript notes of a course of lectures on medicine, delivered in 1841/2, by C. B. J. Williams, one of the leading teachers of his day, there occurs the following passage: 'Diathesis is merely a disposition to a disease, it gives no idea of its cause.' The word diathesis is not to be found in the indexes of the great majority of English text-books of Medicine, published during the last fifty years. In the *New English Dictionary*, in a volume (D), which was published in 1897, diathesis is defined as 'a permanent (hereditary or acquired) condition of the body, which renders it liable to certain special diseases or affections; a constitutional predisposition or tendency'. The words printed in brackets (as in the original) raise a highly controversial question, and clearly reflect the teaching of Jonathan Hutchinson.

Undoubtedly a diathesis has always been thought of by the great majority of physicians in this country, as an inborn, and usually inherited predisposition.

In the French schools, on the other hand, there early became manifest a tendency to apply the name to predisposition to the manifestations of a disease, rather than to the disease as such.

Thus, he who developed a succession of abscesses was regarded as the subject of a purulent diathesis, he who bled frequently of a haemorrhagic diathesis, a name which is still occasionally applied to the disease haemophilia. Bazin enumerated a number of such diatheses, calcareous, saccharine, fatty, fibrinous, and the like.

[35]

On the other hand there were always members of the French school who did not share the prevalent views, and amongst them Roche,[1] as the quotation at the head of this chapter shows.

Towards the middle of the nineteenth century the conceptions had become narrowed down and assumed more definite form. A diathesis came to be looked upon as a comparatively slight deviation from normality, a 'peculiarity of health' as Hutchinson[2] called it, or in the words of Germain Sée:[3] 'Cet état intermédiaire qui n'est pas encore la maladie, mais qui n'est déjà plus la santé parfaite.'

Just as in a mushroom-bed a hidden, underground mycelium throws up mushrooms here and there, and from time to time, so the diathesis is regarded as latent, but its presence is revealed by the manifestations to which it gives rise from time to time. It is easy to see how largely the phenomena of gout, which has always been regarded as the typical diathetic disease, have been instrumental in shaping this conception.

In Nysten's Dictionary, published in 1858, diathesis was defined as a general disposition, in virtue of which an individual is affected by several local affections of the same nature, and Trousseau[4] quotes, with approval, a similar definition in the dictionary of Littré and Robin.

---

[1] *Dict. de Méd. et Chir. Prat.*, 1831, vi. 298.
[2] *The Pedigree of Disease*, 1884, p. 71.
[3] *Leçons de Pathologie expérimentale. Généralités*, p. xiii.
[4] *Clinical Medicine—New Sydenham Society Translation*, iv. 358.

Chomel,[1] writing in 1856, was more explicit. He defined a diathesis as a disposition in virtue of which several organs, or several points in the economy, are, simultaneously or in succession, the seats of affections, spontaneous in their development and identical in their nature, although they may present themselves under different aspects.

On this side of the Channel such views met with more ready acceptance in Edinburgh than in the London schools. Amongst the Edinburgh professors was Thomas Laycock, a man deeply interested in the constitutional aspects of disease, and who instilled into many of his pupils a share of his own enthusiasm. Amongst these was Jonathan Hutchinson, a man of remarkable ability and immense clinical experience, who exercised a profound influence upon medical thought in London, and indeed over a far wider area. When we recall his oral teaching, or read his writings, we realize how his ideas outstripped the knowledge of his day, and how he fell into errors on that account. In his often quoted lectures, published under the title of 'The Pedigree of Disease', Hutchinson expressed views which were in complete accord with those of Trousseau and Chomel. For him diathesis was 'any condition of prolonged peculiarity of health, giving proclivity to definite forms of disease'. He spoke of it as 'a disease which lasts a lifetime, which may be active at times and latent at times, and which may be handed on to another

[1] *Pathologie Générale*, 4th ed., 1856, p. 92.

[37]

generation'. In another place he wrote of a diathesis as little more than an extremely chronic disease.

Obviously those who held such views had moved far away from the conception of adiathesis* as a mere predisposition to a malady. They did not regard it as of necessity an inborn peculiarity, and indeed, both Trousseau and Hutchinson admitted that syphilis†ful-filled all the requirements of their definitions.

Although such conceptions made no wide appeal in this country nor indeed outside France, they did in fact constitute a step forward. As Germain Sée wrote: 'La disposition est un mot pour masquer notre ignorance', and the most that can be said for the word predisposi-tion is that it states the fact that some are more liable than others to this or that disease. Trousseau, Chomel, Hutchinson, on their part were feeling their way to-wards a conception of something much more than a mere word, to that of an underlying state to which the liability is due. Just as W. H. Walshe,[1] another Edinburgh graduate, in a lecture delivered as early as in 1855, pictured the diathetic maladies as 'apparently generated and sustained by an intrinsic blood-poison resulting from some perversion of the nutritive pro-cesses of the individual'.

Probably no explanation has come nearer to the truth, but many years elapsed before the progress of bio-chemistry provided it with a firm foundation, and the diathetic diseases included in Walshe's list form a very

[1] *Med. Times and Gaz.*, 1855, xxxi. 613.

* *adiathesis*   A printer's error noticed by Garrod, but let stand.

† *syphilis*   It is easy to appreciate now that inborn predispositions to disease might have been considered unimportant at the time of Garrod's writing, when pleiotropic extrinsic causes of disease, such as syphilis, were still very prevalent.

miscellaneous collection. Amongst them were infective maladies, such as tuberculosis and leprosy, a number of cutaneous disorders, leukaemia and cyanaemia, oxaluria, phosphaturia and a deficiency disease, scurvy. Obviously theory had quite outstripped fact.

A further development, which had its origin in the French school, was the conception of what might be called the larger diatheses, arthritic, strumous, dartrous and the like, under which headings were grouped sets of maladies, often with little obvious affinity save that they are apt to occur in association.

Of such diatheses arthritism proved the most viable, and has played a large part in the teachings of the French school.

Debove,[1] writing in 1903, acknowledged that the term arthritism, in so common use in France, was little heard beyond her borders, and was wont to surprise foreigners. He described it as embracing things true and things false; and as including a number of maladies which do not involve the joints, but have a certain affinity to gout. Amongst these he mentioned glycos-uria, renal colic and obesity. Debove added that the category could be extended indefinitely according to the views of the enumerator.

Mention should be made of another view of arthri-tism, of which Hanot was an adherent, which looked upon it as an impairment of the power of resistance of the fibrous tissues in general, producing a liability to the

[1] 'Étiologie de la Goutte', *Arch. Gén. de Méd.*, 1903, i. 865.

conditions which Luff includes under the name of fibrositis. This suggestion has a special interest in connexion with the tissue defects, or abiotrophies, presently to be discussed.

The doctrine of arthritism reached its culminating point with the appearance, in 1882, of Bouchard's well-known book, *Maladies par Rallentissement de la Nutrition*. Not only did Bouchard present, in clearly set out sequence, the arguments in support of the existence of an arthritic diathesis, and the inclusion of certain morbid events under that name; but also he took a long step in advance of his predecessors, in that he was the first to attempt to explain the association together of the several members of the arthritic complex by assigning to them a definite, common cause, namely a slackening of the metabolic processes.

Although Bouchard was not the first to suggest an underlying chemical basis of predisposition, he was the first to suggest a chemical defect of a tangible kind, instead of a quite intangible factor behind a group of kindred or apparently kindred maladies. The discovery of uric acid in the blood of gouty people, which opened a new field of clinical chemistry, had been made some thirty years previously, and chemical theories readily suggested themselves in connexion with other diseases.

Bouchard's monograph, which appeared to set the doctrine of arthritism upon so scientific a basis, produced a deep impression at the time of its publication, and his views gained wide acceptance, both in his own

[40]

and other countries. Nevertheless his fundamental conception proved to be ill-founded, and the progress of biochemistry has taught us that matters are far less simple than he supposed.

The work of Emil Fischer, and his successors, which has revealed the structure of the molecules of the proteins, and similar investigations of the other main constituents of living organisms, together with a better understanding of the metabolic processes of which the tissues are the seats, have taught us that the metabolic processes are carried out step by step. The huge protein molecule is not burnt as a whole, but its component aminoacids are dealt with individually, along different lines, and by specialized enzymes. Only the hormones secreted by certain endocrine glands, and notably by the thyroid, have the power of regulating metabolism as a whole. A general damping down of the metabolic forces may explain some of the phenomena of myxoedema and cretinism, but cannot account for the troubles grouped together by Bouchard under the heading of arthritism.

The doctrines of diathesis occupy a very small place in German medical literature. In 1911 the subject was discussed at a meeting of the Kongress für innere Medizin,[1] and in the course of that discussion Wilhelm His said: 'We understand by diathesis an individual, inborn, and often inherited state, in virtue of which physiological stimuli produce abnormal reactions; and condi-

---

[1] *Verhandl. d. deutsch Kong. für inn. Med.*, 1911, xxviii. 15–106.

tions of life which are harmless to the majority of members of the race bring about morbid states.' His added that diatheses differ in degree in different individuals, and at different times, and that their lower limits merge imperceptibly into the normal. Such a definition approaches very closely to those usually given of idiosyncrasy,[*] and von Behring, who put forward a similar definition, distinguished diathesis from idiosyncrasy in that the former implies sensitiveness to stimuli of various kinds, whereas the stimulus which evokes an idiosyncrasy is of some one definite kind.

A definition recently put forward by R. J. Ryle [1] supplies a bridge between the older and newer knowledge.[†] Ryle suggests that we should think of a diathesis as 'a transmissible variation in the structure or function of tissues rendering them peculiarly liable to react in a certain way to certain extrinsic stimuli', and adds that 'not all who acquire the disease have the diathesis, but those who have the diathesis are more likely to acquire the disease than those who have not'.

This brings us round full circle to the original notion of a predisposition to a malady.

It was the coming of bacteriology, which supplies in the bacteria definite, concrete agents of disease, attacking the organism from without, that caused interest in diathesis and kindred conceptions to flag. Attention became concentrated upon the seed rather than upon the

[1] 'Physical Type and Reactions to Disease', *Guy's Hosp. Gaz.*, 1926, xl. 546.

[*] *idiosyncrasy*   A review of *The inborn factors in disease* (*Lancet* 1932) called it a 'pregnant little book' and singled out Ryle's definition of diathesis as among the best.

[†] *A Definition* et seq.   Ryle's definition of diathesis looks very like that which is called 'genetic susceptibility' today. By 'the transmissible variation' is meant, presumably, inherited variation. Note that the cause of disease in this

soil, and it was almost forgotten that there are maladies which owe their origin to no such external invaders.

Those inborn factors which must needs be studied at the bedside were relegated to a back place, and received but scanty attention either from teachers or students. The word diathesis, around which so many controversies had centred, was relegated to the dust-heap of obsolete terms. Only here and there a voice crying in the wilderness pleaded for a hearing for the older views.

But it is not in the laboratory alone that scientific work can be carried out, and once again the pendulum, having reached the limit of its swing, has entered upon its return journey. The inborn factors in disease are once more attracting attention, especially in Germany and Austria, but the word constitution has taken the place of diathesis and its contemporary terms. Such works as those of Julius Bauer,[1] very storehouses of information on this subject, bear witness to the depth as well as to the extent of the reawakened interest.

Constitutional Clinics have been established in various centres, notably in New York, Berlin, and Turin, in which valuable investigations are being carried on by anthropometric and other methods.

In our own country the reawakened interest has been less vocal, but the attention which the constitutional aspects of disease are attracting is greater than the

[1] *Die Konstitutionelle Disposition zu inneren Krankheiten*, 3rd ed., 1924. *Vorlesungen über allgemeine Konstitutions- und Vererbungslehre*, 2nd ed., 1923.

definition is an extrinsic stimulus. Hence, Garrod was apparently considering multifactorial disease in this application of the definition and not an inborn error of metabolism. The argument revolving around cause—intrinsic predisposition, extrinsic stimulus, one or other, or both—surfaces clearly in the following three paragraphs.

scantiness of its literature might lead one to suppose. Undoubtedly the interest is growing, and year by year the need to study the part which the patient plays in connexion with his maladies is emphasized by fresh spokesmen, amongst whom A. F. Hurst, J. A. Ryle, Langdon Brown, and Maitland Ramsay [1] call for special mention.

The word constitution has a much wider significance than had diathesis, and predisposition to disease is only one facet of the subject. The constitution of a man is the sum of all his qualities and all his peculiarities. It embraces the colour of his hair and eyes, the shape of his head and limbs and features, his functional peculiarities, physical and chemical, and the mental and psychological features which take so large a part in shaping his relations to his environment. Each and all of these factors have a share in rendering him more or *less* liable to a disease than his fellows. Relative natural immunity [*] is, indeed, no less important than morbid predisposition.

Moreover, the constitution of the patient plays a very important part in *shaping* the diseases from which he suffers. The picture of a malady represents the reaction of the patient, his protest against the attack and his devices for repulsing it.

Until recently the subject has always been approached from the standpoint of the would-be healer rather than

---

[1] A. F. Hurst, *Brit. Med. Journ.*, 1927, i. 823, 866; J. A. Ryle, loc. cit., sub. 9; W. Langdon Brown, *Brit. Med. Journ.*, 1930, i. 525; A. Maitland Ramsay, *Glasgow Medical Journal*, 1927, viii. 65.

[*] *Relative natural immunity* Garrod was interested in both the adaptive and disadaptive human traits. His thinking was both biological and medical.

that of the naturalist who studies man and his disorders
from the point of view of biology. This one-sided
approach has coloured all the ideas which were advanced,
from time to time, concerning constitutional tendencies,
temperaments, and diatheses. The ideas which under-
lay those terms originated, for the most part, in times
when many of the concepts of modern science were as
yet unformed, when little was known of the laws of
heredity, when the theory of evolution had not yet taken
form, and when such entities as chromosomes, hormones, vitamins, and antitoxins were not yet dreamed of.

In order that we may get further it will be necessary
to re-lay all the foundations of our subject by the light of
the newer knowledge. When so doing many cherished
notions and some time-honoured terms will have to be
discarded, whilst many new facts will need to be taken
into account. This is what is being attempted in the
constitutional clinics and elsewhere, and it is the purpose of this essay to try to sketch the useful lines of
approach to a better understanding of the parts played
by inborn factors in connexion with morbid states.

The essay is divided into two parts. In the first
section the fundamental studies upon which the reconstructed edifice will need to be built up will be reviewed
briefly. Firstly, the meaning of the terms health and
disease need to be considered.

Next, the bearing upon medical problems of recent
advances of biochemistry will be discussed, and after
that the influence of the theory of evolution upon

medical thought; and finally the bearings upon medical questions of the modern theories of heredity. In the second section an attempt will be made to apply the newer knowledge to the problems presented by individual groups of maladies.

In the first place the relation of disease to physical structure will be considered under two heads, namely, the liability of persons of different builds, features, and general conformations to develop particular maladies, and secondly, the influence of structural anomalies and deviations from type, indirectly predisposing to disease. A chapter will be devoted to that most interesting group of hereditary maladies the tissue defects, or abiotrophies as Gowers called them; some of which do not manifest their presence for years after birth. In another chapter will be discussed the influence of deviations from the average chemical structure and chemical life of the tissues in predisposing to, and shaping the manifestations of, some diseases.

The inborn factors in infective maladies will call for consideration; and lastly the idiosyncrasies, the remarkable sensitivities of some individuals to influences which have no obvious ill effects upon the vast majority of the members of the human race. These range from idiosyncrasies with regard to particular pollens or animal emanations, to grave allergic diseases, such as asthma.

The several conclusions reached and inferences to be drawn, will be summed up in an epilogue.

It may appear to some that the subjects here dis-

cussed, however attractive from the scientific standpoint, have but little bearing upon the practice of
medicine,* and few important lessons for those whose
work lies in the sick-room and hospital ward.

It may even be suggested that although the study of
the constitutional aspects of disease has been, to a large
extent, relegated to the background during the last
half-century, there has been, during that same half-
century, an unparalleled advance of both medicine and
surgery. But it must not be forgotten that, in so far as
those advances are in the field of preventive medicine
and aseptic surgery, they are only in a minor degree
concerned with inborn factors; for so long as the individual is sheltered from attack, his powers of resistance are not called into play.

Another great line of advance has been the application of laboratory methods to the solution of clinical
problems; whereas it is in the ward rather than in the
laboratory that the importance of inborn factors is to be
appreciated. The clinical worker relies largely upon
what may be called his clinical insight; a quality which
is purely innate, but which has been developed more
and more as the outcome of accumulated experience.
The family doctor has watched many of his patients
from their birth onwards, and perhaps their parents
before them. They trust him because, as they say, 'he
knows their constitutions'.

The medical man trains himself or has been trained,
by the example of those who taught him, to recognize

* *little bearing upon*   When a disease type has both intrinsic and extrinsic
forms of cause, the relative importance of the intrinsic causes increases when
the extrinsic causes have decreased. Medical practice in Garrod's time was
overshadowed by diseases with extrinsic causes.

the qualities and individual needs of his patients. He realizes that each is an individual,[*] and not merely a member of the human race. The task of the practitioner is far more than to apply the knowledge supplied to him from the laboratories; he does not merely ask himself, or look to his text-books to tell him, what is good for pneumonia, but calls upon his experience to guide him as to how he may best help the particular patient to come through his attack of pneumonia with the least possible damage.

Wittingly or unwittingly, the practitioner of medicine is constantly engaged in the study of constitutions and predispositions, and of reactions to environment. He must, throughout his active life, be a student of the inborn as well as of the external factors in disease.

---

* *each is an individual*   Garrod here differentiates two kinds of individuality; that which goes with membership in the human race and many other classes, and that which pertains to each person's uniqueness. It is one of Garrod's most important distinctions that he thought in terms of individual uniqueness, while others were preoccupied by the characteristics of classes. The tendency to overlook the details of individual uniqueness in 'cases' of diseases still prevails in modern medicine.

PART I

THE BASIC PRINCIPLES OF PRE-DISPOSITION

I

HEALTH AND DISEASE

Men are called healthy in virtue of an inborn capacity to easy resistance to those unhealthy influences that may ordinarily arise; unhealthy in virtue of the lack of that capacity.—ARISTOTLE, *Categoriae*, viii. (trans. Edgehill).

THE living man may be compared to an aviator upon war service, whose safety depends upon a number of different factors. As he flies over the enemy's lines he is a target for shot and shell, is at the mercy of wind and weather; and his life depends upon his own alertness and resource, upon supply of fuel and of oil for lubrication, and upon the efficiency of all parts of his machine. So too we, as we go through life, are assailed by bacteria and protozoa; our well-being is at the mercy of our environment, and depends upon climate and food-supplies. Moreover, if our tissues are not of the first class of their kind, they show, prematurely, signs of wear and tear.

As Aristotle clearly recognized, what we call health is no mere quiescent state, but a condition of unstable equilibrium,* maintained by a continual struggle. His definition, with its so modern ring, has much in com-

3482   D

* *condition of unstable equilibrium* W. B. Cannon's *The wisdom of the body* (Cannon 1932) is about homeostasis. It was published one year after Garrod's *Inborn factors*. One could say that diathesis is homeostasis on the verge of trouble.

[49]

mon with some of the most recent definitions of health and disease. Thus, George Draper,[1] in his book on *The Human Constitution*, defines disease as 'the expression of the reaction between a complex set of external agents and an equally complex organism striving to survive in the midst of them', and F. W. Andrewes,[2] who speaks of the healthy body as not only perfectly adjusted to its surroundings, but capable of adjusting itself, within reasonable limits, to a rapidly changing environment, defines disease as a condition in which the body has fallen, in greater or less degree, out of harmony with its surroundings.

Still more recently, H. D. Rolleston[3] spoke of disease as 'the mental picture of the manifest reactions of a living organism in response to harmful factors, whether derived from outside the body or arising internally'.

These recent definitions all avoid the error against which that great teacher, Thomas Watson,[4] warned his hearers, in a lecture delivered almost a century ago. He bade them avoid 'the strange mistake, too often made or imputed, of regarding disease as a thing, or (as the phrase goes) a "separate entity" by which the body is possessed and damaged—something which can be contemplated as apart from the body, which it may invade'. Watson added that, 'for the most part, disease consists in some derangement, suspension or perversion of the

[1] *Human Constitution*, 1924, p. 222.
[2] *Lancet*, 1926, i. 1075.　　　[3] *Brit. Med. Journ.*, 1929, i. 281.
[4] *Lectures on the Principles and Practice of Physic*, 5th ed., 1871, i. 6.

continuous, normal, nutritive mutation and renewal of the bodily tissues.'

Nevertheless, teachers of medicine and authors of text-books still find themselves obliged to treat, in sequence, of series of discrepant pictures called diseases; as if maladies were all of a kind, and capable of being classified into systematic groupings,* corresponding to the genera and species of plants and animals.

How else, indeed, could they present their subject to their hearers and readers? As Wilhelm His [1] pointed out in a recent Rectorial Address, many morbid pictures recur over and over again with only trifling variations, and to disregard such groupings would result in chaos. Nevertheless, the morbid pictures must not be looked upon as occupying rigidly defined compartments, but rather as merging into each other.

Even if an attempt be made to reach a more scientific classification of diseases by grouping together all the effects of invasion of the organism by some special bacterion† such as the tubercle bacillus—a method for which there is much to be said from the standpoint of the bacteriologist—from the standpoint of the clinical worker nothing will be gained by the association, under a single heading, of pictures so widely different as those of pulmonary tuberculosis, tuberculous meningitis, spinal caries, and Addison's disease.

There are similar objections to the assembling, under one heading, of all the morbid effects of the continued

[1] *Ueber die natürliche Ungleichheit der Menschen.* Berlin, 1928.

* *classified into* The medical curriculum still fosters systems of taxonomy as if most diseases were entities imposed upon patients (the 'ontological' view). Garrod's view embraces the 'physiological' concept of disease; he asks why a particular person might be susceptible to a particular disorder (then see Garrod's next-but-one paragraph).

† *bacterion* Garrod notes that bacterion is the correct singular (letter of 25.03.1931 to Publisher) but admits 'bacterium' is the customary 'much less euphonious' usage.

administration of such a poison as lead or alcohol. The clinical pictures of the gastro-intestinal, cerebral, and peripheral-neuritic effects of lead poisoning, and that of saturnine gout, differ so widely amongst themselves, that if they were not known to have a common origin they would be looked upon as distinct maladies.

Indeed, the symptom-complexes which we call diseases have, for the most part, little in common beyond the facts that they constitute departures from the average standard of health, and tend to bring about, sooner or later, conditions incompatible with the survival of their subjects. These two aspects lie behind the various designations of disease. The Greek and Latin terms νόσος and *morbus* convey the idea of fatality, whereas the more modern terms such as ailment, illness, *maladie*, and the word disease itself, point rather to the discomfort entailed than to danger to life.

So greatly have our notions regarding disease been influenced by the progress of bacteriology, and by all that that science has taught us, that we are in danger of forgetting that not all maladies have their origin outside the body, nor are due to invasion by bacterion, protozoon or virus. The man plays a very important part in connexion with his diseases, and to quote Hippocrates:[1] 'As to the manner of diseases, upon inquiry it will be found, that some are born with us.'

Indeed in all diseases there are both internal and ex-

[1] *De Humoribus*, § 12. (*Hippocrates: Upon Air, Water and Situation*, trans. by Francis Clifton, 1734, p. 41.)

ternal factors. Sometimes the one and sometimes the other is the more conspicuous.

Each one of us is exposed, during every day of his life, to unhealthy influences to which he has some inborn capacity of resistance, but the degree of that capacity varies widely, even amongst individuals who pass as healthy. It is, moreover, a discriminative capacity, different individuals being resistent to different kinds of attack.[*]

On the other hand, there are many of us who possess latent defects of structure or function, inborn and for the most part inherited, which are apt to be revealed, sooner or later, by the effects produced by external influences which are innocuous to the average man. Upon some of the subjects of such defects slight injuries, upon others exposure to bright light or to extremes of temperature, exert a deleterious action. For some individuals those trifling traumata which go to make up the wear and tear of daily life, are apparently the provoking causes of grave disorders.

As the pictures upon the walls of an art gallery are by a variety of artists and of widely different kinds; some portraits, others landscapes, others again subject pictures, and some studies of still life; so the clinical pictures which we call diseases differ markedly amongst themselves, and are indeed the products of different kinds of processes. Nevertheless, some of them fall into groups which have much in common. Of such groups the infectious fevers offer the most obvious examples; they form a natural family of maladies.

* *degree of ... capacity; and, discriminative capacity* Here Garrod distinguishes two kinds of susceptibility: on the one hand, liability or resistance in each person to the adverse effects of different agents or experiences and, on the other, gradations of liability to each such experience among different people. His appreciation of this property, and its implication of fine resolution in the degree of resistance (or susceptibility) has its modern counterpart, for example, in the combinatorial sorting of somatic cell genes to make antibodies and T-cell receptors.

In the infective diseases a morbific agent, a bacterion, a virus, or a protozoon, enters the body from
without, and in so doing gives rise to trouble. In such
cases the external factor is something concrete, which
may be studied outside the body; but daily experience
teaches that there are also internal factors at work, that
there is such a thing as a natural liability to, and
a natural immunity against infective diseases. Moreover, it is the human subject rather than the specific
micro-organism which shapes the syndromes or clinical pictures by which such diseases are recognized;
although a similar response follows a specific bacterial
infection in different subjects. The severity of the
attack, although in part controlled by the virulence
of the invading germ, is also a measure of the resist-
ing power of the organism, its natural or acquired
immunity; in other words by the efficiency of its defensive mechanisms.

If we could watch from the air the landing of a hostile
force upon our shores, we should witness the disturbances thereby induced in the invaded area, the muster-
ing of troops for the defence, and the evacuation of the
inhabitants. These operations, which would fill the fore-
front of the picture, would represent the reaction of the
people attacked. So also, in the case of an acute infection, the clinical picture shows the marshalling and
organization of the defence of the body.

Even fever may be regarded as a beneficial rather
than a harmful process, so long as the thermotaxic

[54]

mechanism remains well under control, and the temperature does not rise to a level which is gravely deleterious
to the tissues. To quote Andrewes[1] once more, a
bacterial infection does not always give rise to morbid
happenings, as the symptom-free carriers of pathogenic
bacteria show, only when the body begins to defend itself against attack does trouble arise: 'It is an evil that
a tissue should become inflamed and that the body temperature should rise in an acute infection; but it is a
lesser evil than that the infecting agent should overrun
the body unchecked by any antagonistic mechanism.'

Individual cases of any particular disease, infective
or other, are not exactly alike, as are the prints pulled
from a lithographic block; they resemble rather the
drawings made from the same model by individual
members of a drawing class. The differences between
one case and another are often very slight, but they are
familiar to all who practise medicine. By no means all
such differences are due to the constitutional peculiarities of the patients; in the infective maladies, as has been
mentioned, the virulence of the pathogenic organism
plays an important part, and the clinical picture presented may be modified profoundly by the severity
and distribution of local lesions resulting from the
disease.

On the other hand, factors inherent in the patient undoubtedly play important parts in modifying the syndrome observed; as is witnessed by the conspicuous

[1] Loc. cit., sub. 2.

differences between cases of the same infective malady
in children and adults respectively. No better example
can be quoted than that of rheumatic fever. In the child
the greater frequency and severity of the cardiac accidents, and the frequency of chorea and nodules, together with the comparative insignificance of the articular lesions, which are so conspicuous in adults, give to
the syndrome a special stamp. As other instances may
be cited the different distribution of the local manifestations of tuberculous and pneumococcal infections in
children and adults respectively. The influence of sex is
much less obvious; but apart from obvious examples of
sex-linked inheritance, there is evidence of relative immunities and liabilities in males and females respectively.
Draper,[1] in a recent book gives statistics of the incidence
of diseases in the two sexes, for many of which no obvious
explanation offers itself. We do not know why pneumonia should be much commoner in males, and purpura
haemorrhagica in females. Some such differences may
be ascribable to occupations, and some to secondary
sexual causes.

Another well-defined group of maladies, widely
different in their outer aspects, but akin in their origins,
are the so-called deficiency diseases. In them instead of
an invading micro-organism the main external cause is
lack of a vitamin*; if indeed a negative factor can properly
be described as an external cause.

It is inevitable that an organism which depends upon

[1] *Disease and the Man*, 1930, p. 108 et seq.

* *lack of a vitamin* F. Gowland Hopkins (viz. Needham 1962) a colleague
of Garrod, was awarded a Nobel Prize for his share in the discovery of
'accessory food substances' (now called vitamins). Deficient intake of a
specific vitamin had been shown to cause specific disease types in animals and
man. Examples suggesting predisposition to adverse consequences of vitamin
deficiency are mentioned on pp. 33 and 34 of *Inborn factors*.

supplies from without must experience serious troubles if any of those supplies are withheld; as witness the phenomena of anoxaemia, culminating in suffocation, and those of starvation of various degrees; but in the diseases under discussion the dietetic errors are much more subtle. The vitamins, which might be described as exogenous hormones, cannot be reckoned as foodstuffs, but exert a profound influence over nutrition.

The vitamin C, which is soluble in water, is contained in foods which avert or cure scurvy; and when it is lacking the tissues are rendered unduly vulnerable to slight injuries, and injuries, slight or severe, play the chief parts in determining the occurrence and distribution of haemorrhages in scorbutic subjects. In the same way the fat-soluble vitamin D is concerned with bone and tooth formation, and lack of it induces rickets; but as is now known, the organism is not wholly dependent upon supplies of that vitamin from without; for it can be formed from ergosterol in the skin, by irradiation with light or ultra violet rays.

As to the influence of personal factors in deficiency diseases, clinical evidence, and especially that derived from work in children's hospitals, suggests strongly that some individuals are much better able than others to carry on despite shortages of vitamins.

That some infants develop scurvy upon diets which others can take with impunity, or even upon a diet which appears hardly open to criticism, is a matter of

common experience, whereas other infants appear to be
relatively immune. McCarrison,[1] who bases his opinion
mainly upon experimental feeding of animals, speaks
confidently of the existence of individual predispositions to deficiency diseases. He holds that 'the quanti-
ties of vitamins necessary for the harmonious regulation of the metabolic processes vary with the individual
and his rate of metabolism'. Moreover, he found that
different organs of the body have their individual
liabilities, as also has the same organ in different individuals, and concluded that 'idiosyncrasy, whether of
individual subjects or of individual organs, is an important factor in determining the onset and the manifestations of deficiency disease'. That the stage of development of the patient's tissues plays an important
part in shaping the clinical picture, is evidenced by the
difference between infantile scurvy with its subperio-
steal haemorrhages, and the same malady as met with
in adults.

In a third group might be included what may be
called the allergic diseases, such as asthma, at least in
some of its forms, and angio-neurotic oedema; but this
group is not clearly defined, for allergic phenomena play
conspicuous parts in a variety of maladies, including the
exanthemata. The external cause often appears quite
inadequate to bring about such striking results as are
seen, in not a few cases, to follow the inhalation of the
pollen of grass or the exhalation of a particular kind of

[1] *Studies in Deficiency Disease*, 1921, p. 40.

animal. The internal factors, on the other hand, are
conspicuous, and that, in many cases at least, the hypersensitivity is inborn is shown by its appearance in
successive generations of a family.

Athwart such lines of classification runs a system of
grouping of diseases according to the organs or parts
which they affect, and with such groupings neither
medical teachers nor writers have been able to dispense.
A peculiarly interesting group of such syndromes is
that resulting from lesions of the endocrine glands.*
Just as the several glands have widely different functions, the syndromes which result from suppression
of their functions, or from excessive secretion of their
hormones, are of diverse kinds. No more clearly defined
diseases exist than exophthalmic goitre and myxoedema,
acromegaly and Addison's disease; but seeing that the
functional derangement may be of any degree, the textbook descriptions of these maladies are obviously based
upon extreme examples. There are all grades of hypo-
and hyper-thyroidism. Although in most instances the
underlying morbid process in an endocrine disease is of
the same nature, as in the case of the adrenal lesions of
Addison's disease, which are almost always tuberculous,
there is no necessary connexion between the syndrome
due to error of glandular function and the nature of the
glandular lesions.

There is an obvious analogy between the maladies
due to lack of a hormone, and the deficiency diseases,
but the analogy must not be pressed too far. L. J.

---

* *endocrine glands* The excitement associated, in Garrod's time, with
advances in the new discipline of endocrinology is apparent in *The inborn
factors of disease*. Garrod considered hormones to be important components of
metabolic regulation— or 'homeostasis' as it was called later by Cannon
(1932). It is known now that gene expression can be modified by hormones.

Harris and T. Moore[1] have brought forward some evidence of the existence of a vitamin balance comparable to the balance of the endocrine glands which constitutes the great regulator mechanism of the bodily processes.

More crude effects are produced in a variety of morbid conditions, by pressure on ducts of such glands as the liver or pancreas, or upon neighbouring blood-vessels or nerve-trunks. As an example may be cited the often-repeated clinical picture of carcinoma of the head of the pancreas.

A large and most characteristic group of morbid pictures is provided by the diseases of the nervous system. From such pictures the skilled neurologist can often localize with accuracy the seats of lesions of the brain or spinal cord, and experience often enables him to deduce the nature of the lesion to which the syndrome is due. No more striking example of such a syndrome can be quoted than that of tabes dorsalis, which is now known to be a manifestation of syphilitic infection.

Amongst nervous diseases there are some which are strongly hereditary, but in which there is little evidence of the working of any external causative factor. Of such pseudo-hypertrophic muscular dystrophy offers a good example.

The syndrome due to a local lesion will obviously vary according to the extent of the lesion; as is seen in

[1] Harris and Moore, *Biochemical Journal*, 1929, xxiii. 114.

the early extension and later contraction of the paralysis produced by poliomyelitis.

It is obvious that many different factors are concerned in the production of the various morbid pictures which differ so widely in their characters; and that the factors which predispose an individual to one malady may be wholly different from those which predispose him to another. Nor is it to be wondered at that no satisfactory system of classification of diseases has been evolved, seeing that the items to be classified are, in many instances, not really comparable; as Thomas Watson said, they are not entities.

Nor is it to be wondered at that wholly different views have been, and are, entertained as to what is entitled to be called the cause of a disease, and these differences of opinion extend even to the infective maladies. Whereas to some it appears obvious that the cause of such a malady is the infecting organism, and around this tenet modern medicine has, to a large extent, taken shape, there are others who maintain that the cause of pneumonia is not the pneumococcus, but rather a state of the tissues of the individual infected, which brings about a response of a characteristic kind to the specific invasion.

Those who are interested in such discussions will find the conflicting views, and the arguments upon which they rest, ably set out in the writings of Lubarsch, Julius Bauer, F. Kraus, Hueppe and Martius [1] amongst

[1] Lubarsch, *Deut. med. Wchnschr.*, 1922, xlviii. 787, 1025; Bauer, J.,

others. To some of us it will seem that the disputants are beating the air; that there is right upon both sides, and that both are wrong if they claim that any single factor is entitled to be spoken of as *the cause* of any malady. We may hold, with Lubarsch, that it is misleading to assert that the tubercle bacillus is the cause of tuberculosis, and may prefer to say that the entry into, and multiplication of tubercle bacilli in a predisposed body is the cause of that disease.

The two factors, the soil and the seed, the external and the internal, must both be taken into account if we are to form any adequate conception of the nature and causation of any disease. The relative importance and prominence of the two factors vary very widely; but whilst on the other hand, the constitutional factor cannot safely be ignored when discussing the causation of pneumonia, it is equally necessary not to leave out of account, when discussing the causation of haemophilia, the slight injury which may have started a fatal haemorrhage.

It is permissible to suppose that, as in the production of those wider departures from the standard of health which receive the name of diseases, both internal and external factors are at work, so also in the causation of those lesser departures, which it is difficult to name or classify, and which may be spoken of as trifling ail-

Die konstitutionelle Disposition zu inneren Krankheiten, 3rd ed., 1924; Kraus, F., *Die allgemeine und spezielle Pathologie der Person*, 1919; Martius, F., *Deut. med. Wchnschr.*, 1918, xliv. 449, 481.

ments, there are internal and external factors concerned of such minor degrees that their presence is hardly recognizable, or fails to be detected by the methods at our disposal.

II

THE CHEMICAL BASIS OF INDIVIDUALITY

The particular chemical type, the particular mode and rate of the chemical changes of tissues, passes from father to son, as the shape of the features passes.—JOHN SIMON. 1876.

IN the preceding sketch of the history of the doctrines of diathesis it was mentioned that, as far back as the middle of the nineteenth century, some writers had suggested that the liabilities of certain individuals to particular diseases might have their origin in disturbances or irregularities of the metabolic processes of the individuals in question. At that time such an explanation was open to the objection that it explained the unknown by the even less known; but although biochemistry has made immense advances since then, the further the matter is investigated the more probable does it appear that the suggestion is justified.

It will be desirable therefore to examine, in this section, the evidence which favours the supposition that our individuality has a chemical basis; for the inborn factors in disease are merely facets of our individuality.*

In our pursuit of this aim it will be necessary to go back as far as the very germinal cells and their chromo-

* . . . *for the inborn factors in disease are merely facets of our individuality.* This phrase encapsulates the book.

somes, into which, in the words of J. B. Leathes,[1] 'were packed, from the beginning, all that pertains, if not to our fate and fortunes, at least to our bodily characteristics, down to the colour of our eyelashes'.

It is hardly possible to imagine the concentration of so many potentialities into structures so minute, unless we suppose that the underlying factors of the various future developments are inherent in the molecules of which the chromosomes are built up. Huxley[2] realized this when he wrote, as long ago as in 1875, that 'to be a teleologist and yet accept evolution it is only necessary to suppose that the original plan was sketched out, that the purpose was foreshadowed, in the molecular arrangements out of which the animals have come'.

In his illuminating Rectorial Address, delivered in Prague in 1896, Huppert[3] argued that chemical differences in the constituents of the germ-cells must determine the attributes of the organisms developed from them. He was one of the first to point out the differences of chemical structure and chemical life of animals of different species; and from such differences he deduced the existence of similar differences in the materials composing the germ-cells from which they spring.

In such a congeries of molecules as a germ-cell, made up, to a large extent, of proteins, nucleoproteins,

---

[1] *British Assoc. Oxford Report*, 1926. Sect. 1, Physiology. Presidential Address, p. 208.
[2] *Life and Letters*, 1900, i. 456.
[3] *Die Erhaltung der Arteigenschaften*. Prague, 1896.

and substances of the lecithin group, which last, being insoluble in water, are the more valuable factors in cell life, there is room for immense variety and for differences not only between species and genera, but also between individuals of a species. In the living organism everything is in flux, there is action everywhere, in the limbs, circulation, and viscera; in the constituent cells of the tissues, in the molecules concerned in the metabolic processes, and even within the very atoms of which the molecules are composed. Every individual differs from every other, there is no rigid line between species and species; no fixed standard of normality and health.

It can hardly be wondered at that, in such an atmosphere of change, numbers of variations from the average occur, nor that some of these are so pronounced as to become conspicuous. It would be more wonderful if it were not so. The departures from the average of the species may be peculiarities either of structure or of function, and there is good reason to believe that even structural diversities have chemical origins.

Mutations, those step-like variations which originate in the germinal cells and are transmissible from generation to generation, may be no more than slight deviations from the average, or may be so conspicuous as to justify their description as occurring *per saltum*. In this connexion Goodrich [1] pictures what happens to a molecule when an atom or an atomic grouping is removed from it, as suggestive of what may occur in the factors of

[1] *Living Organisms*, Oxford, 1924, pp. 85 and 95.

inheritance when a mutation appears. Lenz [1] carries the conception of molecular mutations a step further, and suggests that on any chemico-physical conception of the germ-plasm it is not to be expected that it will be the seat of smooth and continuous change, but rather that it will be altered in successive *steps*, by the removal, or by shifting of the positions of molecular groupings.

One is tempted to venture yet one step further, and to point out that, since in the experimental breeding of *Drosophila* the same mutation is seen to originate over and over again in the species, such a happening may be compared to a chemical reaction in the laboratory, which is repeated as often as the necessary conditions are reproduced.

It is hardly necessary any longer to argue in support of the view that the various genera and species of plants and animals differ in their chemical structure.[*] Not only do we recognize the facts that the fat of a sheep differs in its composition from that of a pig, and that the proteins of an animal of one species act as foreign proteins to animals of another species, but it is also evident that the members of different species differ in what may be called their chemical lives, in that complex of chemical happenings to which we give the name of metabolism.

In the vegetable world such differences are manifested in the pigments of leaves and flowers and the

[1] *Handbuch der normalen und pathologischen Physiologie,* 1926, xvii. 941.

[*] *chemical structure*   In the two preceding paragraphs Garrod refers to the phenomenon of mutation but to what 'molecular grouping' he imputes the event is unclear. The 'chemical structure' referred to here, is of phenotype not genotype.

essential oils to which their scents are due. In the animal world they are borne witness to by specific colourings, by protective secreta, odorous or concealing, less obviously by specific differences of haemoglobins of bile-salts, and of the tissue proteins as revealed by the precipitin test.

Nor can it be doubted that similar, but much more subtle differences than those which distinguish species from species obtain even within the boundaries of the species. Were it not so it would be necessary to picture the existence of specific barriers too rigid to be compatible with the evolution of living forms.

Moreover, there is clear evidence that such differences do actually exist. Some deviations from the chemical type of a species are wide enough to compel attention, such as albinism and certain chemical malformations which will be discussed in a later chapter. Others less conspicuous doubtless escape notice; and others again, still more subtle although often more conspicuous, such as idiosyncrasies to foods and pollens, are still beyond the reach of chemical methods.

Of the differences of this latter class are the remarkable differences in the behaviour of blood when introduced into the circulation of another member of the same species. These phenomena, which are of great practical importance in the practice of transfusion, have attracted much attention in recent years. The blood of human subjects is classed under certain groups according to its behaviour in such circumstances, and the agglutination of the red corpuscles when donor and recipient belong to incompatible groups is attributed to the presence or absence of as yet intangible substances known as agglutinogens and agglutinins.

That membership of the several blood-groups is transmitted from parent to child appears to be well established, and it is suggested that the inheritance follows Mendelian lines. But the groups would appear to represent racial quite as much as individual differences; as would appear from work done upon various races. It would seem that the group known as A is present in higher percentage in the races of Western Europe, and that the percentage of group B tends to increase from west to east.

There is still much to be learned concerning the blood-groups, but it can hardly be doubted that they testify to chemical or physico-chemical differences within the boundaries of the species.

It is the extreme complexity of the molecules of the proteins, which are the essential constituents of all living tissues, that makes it possible to imagine how chemical individuality can exist. Their huge molecules are built up of some twenty or more fractions, each an individual compound, which, being an amino-acid, is capable of acting as an acid and also as a base. To its neighbour on the one side it acts as an acid, to its neighbour on the other side as a base, and so the several constituent fractions are able to hold hands, so to speak, and to form chains and clusters.

The number of possible groupings of the several fractions, in which each fraction is represented only once, is very great indeed, and when it is considered that the proportions of individual amino-acids vary widely and that one or more may be missing from the molecule of any individual protein, it is obvious that the possible combinations and groupings must exceed in numbers even the figures with which astronomers have to deal.

It cannot be doubted that natural selection works through chemical as well as structural modifications, nor that the features in which an organism differs from type are foreshadowed in the molecular complexes of the chromosomes.

In an address delivered in 1926, J. B. Leathes[1] pointed out that all which needs to be premised in order that the whole course of evolution may follow, is the disposition of matter in molecules or aggregates which shall be unstable and immensely variable; and that such matter shall have and retain the power to determine the deposition of other matter in conformity with its own pattern, or with patterns which enable it to exercise such power.

It may be supposed that, as evolution has proceeded, organisms have been produced which differ in chemical structure, as well as in their forms, until the proteins of a group of living things have become so far differentiated. that they behave as foreign proteins towards members

[1] Loc. cit., sub. 1.

even of kindred groups. When that stage has been reached interbreeding will no longer be possible, the species will have been established, and thenceforward its main characteristics will be maintained.

Evidently, as the organism becomes more elaborated there will be ever increasing opportunities of departure from type. As Andrewes puts it, 'a chronometer can suffer from a greater variety of defects than an hour-glass'.

The simpler organisms possess a great power of repairing damaged tissues, but, as evolution proceeds from the single cell to the nations of cells which consti-tute the higher plants and animals, the somatic cells of which their various tissues are built up become specialized for the particular purposes which they are called upon to serve; some to form the skeleton and others muscles; some to produce external and internal secretions, others to ensure the removal of waste materials. In becoming thus specialized the cells lose a part at first, and ultimately almost the whole of their totipotentiality, that power which the primary cells possessed of reconstructing lost parts, and of the more delicate kinds of tissue repair. Such repairs as are still possible are carried out by the wandering cells of the mesenchyme. The reunion of a broken bone, the scar-ring of an abraded surface, the healing of a wound are still possible even for the most highly developed organisms, and hypertrophy or hyperplasia may com-pensate for loss of a part, but in the higher animals a destroyed organ cannot be reproduced, nor a lost limb replaced.

A lizard may grow a new tail of a sort, but in a man who has lost one kidney, the remaining kidney has to enlarge and do the work of two.

Only the germinal cells retain the power to reproduce all the tissues and all the structures of the original organism, and it is in virtue of that power that the reproduction and survival of the species is committed to them. Whatever may happen to the somatic cells affects the individual involved, but not the future of the race. Just as in a bee community the worker bees are specialized for the performance of their appointed tasks, and minister to the fertile queen and her progeny, but have no further share in the propagation of the race, so the somatic cells are specialized to wait upon the needs of the germ-plasm.

Yet the germ-cells are composed of the same kind of materials as the somatic, and although protected from many kinds of injury to which the body-cells are liable they are no more immortal than they. The main difference is that they retain the totipotentiality which the somatic cells have lost. In what that totipotentiality consists we do not know.

There are indications that the germ cells may be altered by certain agencies, such as exposure to X-rays,[*] and that thereby the progeny may be affected; but it is commonly held that to the germinal cells alone is due the transmission of the forms and functional charac-

* *exposure to X-rays* Muller demonstrated the mutagenic effects of X-rays in 1926 and published his work in *Science* (Muller 1927). Garrod could have known of this work but he doesn't refer to it here. He is characteristically sparing of references; there are only 82 in the book.

teristics of the individuals; and if so, we must look to them for the basis of the inborn factors in disease. Each one of us, and each departure from type which he exhibits, may be looked upon as one of Nature's experiments, and the experiment may result in success or failure.

Speaking in 1881, Huxley [1] referring to the normal and typical characteristics of a species said: 'Outside the range of these conditions, the normal course of the cycle of vital phenomena is disturbed; abnormal structure makes its appearance, or the proper character and mutual adjustment of the functions cease to be preserved. The extent and the importance of these deviations from the typical life may vary indefinitely. They may have no noticeable influence on the general well-being of the economy, or they may favour it. On the other hand, they may be of such a nature as to impede the activities of the organism, or even to involve its destruction.'

It is important to bear in mind, in any discussion of constitutional liability to disease, the three possibilities mentioned by Huxley. When approaching the subject from the medical side one is liable to forget the reverse of the picture, the modifications or mutations which are beneficial to the organism. Inborn immunity is no less real than inborn liability to disease. Were there no favourable variations there could be no evolutionary advance. Yet, as will be shown later, it is far more difficult to point to definite examples of favourable

[1] *Internat. Med. Congr. Trans.*, 1881, i. 91.

variations which diminish liability to disease, than to such as favour its development. Moreover, as is remarked by J. B. S. Haldane and Julian Huxley,[1] in a book published recently: 'Mutations most easily detected will usually be those with large and striking effects; and a large change will be likely to throw the animal's organization out of gear. Mutations of small amount which do not throw the machinery out of gear but may even improve it, must also be occurring, but the smaller they are the more difficult will they be to detect.' In other words, the better the adaptation to the environment, the less likely is any change to be for the better.

A new departure may be, at the same time, both beneficial and harmful, but if the good outweighs the evil it will persist.* Thus, when man adopted the erect posture he gave up the hammock-like support of the abdominal viscera, which is a fundamental part of the vertebral plan; and in so doing laid himself open to a variety of minor ills, varicose veins, herniae, and the like; but the gain was far greater than the loss, for it was no less than the mastery of animal nature upon this planet.

It may appear, at first sight, that in this discussion of the basis of individuality an essential difference between variations of form and those of function has been ignored. But, as a matter of fact, the difference is rather apparent than real.

[1] *Animal Biology*, 1927, p. 221.

3482   G

* *A new departure* The compensating advantages of heterozygosity for β-thalassaemia and haemoglobins and of homozygosity for absence of the Fy blood group in the malarial environment were single-gene examples unknown in Garrod's time.

If we are justified in assuming that the representation in the chromosomes of the characteristics of the organism which shall spring from them has a molecular basis, differences of form must themselves have been determined by molecular grouping, in other words, must have a chemical origin.

That chemical factors play a conspicuous part in determining bodily form has been revealed by the study of the endocrine glands and of the hormones which they secrete, two at least of which hormones already take their places amongst known crystalline chemical compounds. It is now generally recognized that the endocrine glands constitute a system of balanced regulators, which control many of the most important processes in the animal body, and through its functions tend to shape its structure. By this balanced control, height and weight, slimness and obesity, and also temperature of the body and blood pressure are kept within the not too narrow limits of what is called normality. But, as in a tug of war there is a swaying to and fro; so, within the bounds of the average, there are many opportunities for variations both small and great.

Not a few writers, notably Keith[1] in this country, L. Bolk[2] in Holland, and Pende[3] in Italy, have emphasized the importance of the role played by the endrocrine glands in connexion with the evolution of the

---

[1] *Huxley Memorial Lecture. Nature*, 1923, cxii. 257.
[2] *Lancet*, 1921, ii. 588.
[3] *Constitutional Inadequacies* (trans.), 1928.

races of mankind, but undoubtedly other influences also are at work. The hormones are essentially regulative rather than inventive. They are fully competent to bring about abnormal stature or hirsuties, but we cannot attribute to them extra digits, nor such other eminently hereditary deformities as claw hand, and must look elsewhere also for the causes of malformations by defect, of structural jobs left unfinished, such as cleft palate and spina bifida.

On the other hand, it can hardly be doubted that the endocrine system plays a most important part in the production of those individual and racial differences of form and feature which are revealed by anthropometry, and of which the association with morbid liabilities, of various kinds, is being studied assiduously in an increasing number of Constitutional Clinics.

Following a completely different line of thought, J. B. Leathes[1] adduces the influence of function, of stress and strain for instance, upon the development of connective tissues. He sees in such influences the exciting causes of a secretion of collagen by certain cells of the connective tissues, and the resultant formation of what may be called a fibrous rigging along the direction of the pull, that is to say of tendons and ligaments. To similar influences may be ascribed the structure of the bones, the distribution of the trabeculae in such a way as to meet the mechanical strain to which the bones are habitually subjected.

[1] Loc. cit., sub. (1).

Starting with such a conception of chemical specificity and chemical individuality as has been sketched out in this chapter, it is not difficult to conceive of the handing down, from parent to child, of those peculiarities of form and function which depend upon the chemical structure of the chromosomes. Nor is it difficult to suppose that natural selection works, through the medium of the mutations which occur and recur from time to time, for the better adaptation of the individual, and through the individual of the race, to the environment in which he lives.

Among the legacies thus handed down from one generation to another are predispositions to certain diseases, or exceptional powers of resistance, which play and have played no unimportant parts in the evolution of the human race.

III

EVOLUTION AND DISEASE

Of all the teeth in the terrible comb with which Nature sorts out the inefficient, disease is one of the most formidable.—F. W. ANDREWES. 1926.[*]

SINCE the days when the older notions of diatheses took form the whole outlook upon biological problems has been profoundly changed by the general acceptance of the theory of evolution; an acceptance which is not impaired by the diversity of views which still persists, as to the mode in which the evolution of living things has come about.

* *Of all the teeth* ... A picturesque description of a process for natural selection in man. Garrod develops the theme in detail in the following pages.

There are, to-day, those who hold that the part played by natural selection has been far less than Darwin supposed, and some who believe that the influence of that factor is almost negligible; despite the fact that when once conceived of, the survival of the fittest is seen to be inevitable. The controversy as to the hereditability of acquired characters still persists, involving, as it does, the vulnerability of the germplasm. The views of Lamarck in modified form, the so-called neo-Lamarckism, have not a few adherents.

Whatever views may be held upon such points, the fact remains that in no discussion of the inborn factors in disease can the evolution of the agents of disease, on the one hand, and that of the methods of defence of the organism, on the other hand, be left out of account.

As to what constitutes fitness to survive, man and Nature do not see eye to eye. As civilization has advanced the protection of the sick and weak as also of those whose mental development gives them but a poor chance in the struggle for existence has become more and more developed. The whole aim of medical art, whether therapeutic or preventive, has been to counteract the laws of Nature.* We certainly would not have it otherwise, and indeed the highest achievements of human thought and of art, are not unfrequently the work of men who are little fitted for the rough and tumble of a life of struggle.

The part played by disease as an agent of evolution, has no doubt been greater in the case of man than of

---

* *aim of medical art* People are prone to ask whether the human gene pool will change in subsequent generations because of treatment of young patients with genetic diseases in present generations. The usual implication of the question is that change will be for the worse.

the lower animals whose lives are in jeopardy every hour, and of civilized man than of his predecessors the pre-historic cave-dwellers. Our early forebears, although exposed to the far more rigorous climate of an ice-age, and lacking the protections which we regard as essential, probably needed such protections less than we do; but they were constantly exposed to the attacks of wild animals against which their weapons were not wholly adequate, and to the assaults of kindred marauding tribes. They had not much opportunity of being sick.

Modern man, on the other hand, leading a far more sheltered life, and perhaps because he does so, is much more likely to succumb to disease—to die in his bed, as the saying is—and he owes his survival far more to the devices of his brain than to the vigour of his arm. Whether, with advance of preventive medicine and hygiene, on the one hand, and the multiplication of motor vehicles on the other, this situation will again become reversed, remains to be seen.

We are apt to forget how closely, as evolution has proceeded, man has become adapted to the calls upon him. The very possibility of protoplasmic life is limited by the effects of temperature upon proteins, and the range is not a wide one, but man is adapted, not only to temperature, but also to the force of gravity at the surface of this planet, to the pressure of the atmosphere and the blending of its constituent gases, to the character and composition of the available foodstuffs. It is not to be wondered at that a deviation from the average on his part is apt to place him at a disadvantage.

On the other hand the normal man is able to adapt himself, in virtue of his regulating mechanisms, to considerable changes in his environment. An obvious example of this is afforded by the survival and well-being of races and individuals, in the tropics or in the polar regions, at the sea-level or on mountain sides, without any conspicuous variation of body temperature.

The relation of evolution to disease has occupied the attention of a number of writers in recent years. Of those, in this country, who have contributed to the discussion the names of G. Adami,[1] F. W. Andrewes,[2] Archdall Reid,[3] and W. J. Collins[4] call for special mention.

In later chapters it will be necessary to speak, in some detail, of special aspects of the subject; here it will suffice to review briefly some of its general aspects.

These fall under three chief headings: In the first place, the means of defence of the organism against attacks from without has obviously been improved by the evolution of ingenious defensive mechanisms. Secondly, in the case of infective maladies the invading organism, whether bacterion or protozoon, has developed improved methods of attack as time has gone on, as was well brought out by Andrewes in his Linacre

---

[1] *Medical Contributions to the Study of Evolution*, 1918.
[2] 'Linacre Lecture. Disease in the Light of Evolution', *Lancet*, 1926, i. 1075.
[3] *Present Evolution of Man*, 1896. [4] *Lancet*, 1920, i. 1059.

Lecture. Thirdly, there can be no question that disease has played, and is playing, a very important part as an instrument of natural selection.

Against maladies which have their origin outside the body, in the introduction into it of protozoa, bacteria, or those still mysterious agents known as filter-passing viruses, and against such diseases as result from administration of poisons of various kinds, there have been evolved protective mechanisms of conspicuous efficiency.

The chemical poisons may be considered first, for they provide the simplest examples, in which fairly simple chemical processes are concerned. The simplest example of all it provided by the measures to counteract acid poisons. The neutralization of the acid by ammonia diverted from metabolism, which has the great merit of sparing the fixed alkalies of the tissues, has been developed in carnivorous animals, including man, but not apparently in herbivora, which having abundance of alkali in their food, are little exposed to acid-poisoning. Another simple, but highly important protective device is the combining of toxic aromatic compounds with sulphates, to form the innocuous aromatic sulphates which are excreted by the kidneys: or with glycine to form the acids of the hippuric group. It appears that only in the case of normal aromatic products of the body chemistry, tyrosin, phenyl-alanin, and tryptophane can the benzene ring be broken in the course of metabolism.

However, it must not be assumed too readily that such mechanisms have been evolved in all cases. It is highly probable that in some instances we have to deal with an unrehearsed chemical reaction. When Baumann administered brom-benzine to a dog the animal excreted a derivative of cystin to which he gave the name of a mercapturic acid. The same happens with all dogs and with other halogen-benzines. Yet it is unlikely that before Baumann's experiment any dog had taken brom-benzine. The mechanism was ready to hand, although the contingency could hardly have been prepared for; just as the organic chemist succeeds in preparing synthetically compounds which have never previously existed, but which assume their correct crystalline form, and exhibit predicted properties. Yet in studying such mechanisms we get a glimpse, behind the scenes, of what may be the inner meaning of what is spoken of as predisposition to disease.

Turning now to the infective* maladies, the protective mechanisms are undoubtedly much more elaborate. The agents of defence are not yet known as definite chemical compounds, but are revealed to us only by single properties. Such are the antitoxins, agglutinins, opsinins, and the like. They are not yet accessible by the ordinary methods of the chemical laboratory. In many instances they are apparently not present in the organism until it is attacked from without, but once acquired they may remain as long-lasting assets of their possessors. Some of them have the power of slaying

3482　　　　　　　　　　H

* *infective* A word Garrod used, and defended (see OED) in discussions with the publisher. Infectious is the usual medical term.

the invaders, whereas others serve as antidotes to their
toxic products.

Apart from these chemical or physico-chemical
methods the organism is able to defend itself by
mobilization of the wandering cells of the mesenchyme.
The phagocytes are rushed to the threatened area; steps
are taken to deal with the invaders by their means and
by hemming them in so as to localize the trouble.

The temperature of the body also is raised to the
optimum level for the altered circumstances. Such is
the picture by which we arecon fronted*if, as Andrewes
does, we look upon fever, and inflammation also, as
part of a well-devised protective scheme.

As to the part which infective diseases have played
in the evolution of the human race it is difficult to bring
forward any definite evidence, but still more difficult
to doubt that that influence has been very great.
Epidemics and pandemics have decimated, and more
than decimated, large populations, as witness the Black
Death in England, and, in a lesser degree, the pandemic
of influenza in 1918. Such outbreaks destroy the strong
as well as the weak, but less highly infectious maladies do
much to weed out the feebler members of the community.

To turn to the other side of the picture it appears to
be certain that populations tend to acquire a considerable degree of protection against those infective diseases
with the infective agents of which they are continually
in contact. The fatal results of the introduction of an
infectious disease, such as measles, into a community

* *arecon fronted*   A printer's error noted by Garrod.

[82]

not previously exposed to it, bear witness to such relative, acquired immunity.

Two explanations of this suggest themselves. On the one hand there can be no doubt that repeated exposure to an infection, even though no attack of the corresponding disease results, does tend to confer a degree of acquired immunity; on the other hand it is difficult to doubt that, as Archdall Reid [1] so strongly maintained, the more susceptible members of a community tend to be eliminated by natural selection, with the result that the surviving population consists mainly of less vulnerable individuals. Naturally this applies only to the maladies which are always with us; a community enjoys no such relative immunity in face of a disease to which it has never previously been exposed.

The other side of the picture need not be discussed here, but should be alluded to. It must not be supposed that the evolutionary processes are concerned for the welfare of the higher animals alone. The bacteria and protozoa which have acquired parasitic habits have their own careers to work out; to ensure their own survival their methods of attack have doubtless been improved, to counter improved methods of defence. We must picture a struggle of conflicting interests, carried on through the ages, perhaps since the dawn of life upon this earth.

But by no means all maladies are due to infective agents, and in some the internal factors play by far the more conspicuous parts. The subject of an unfavourable

[1] Loc. cit.

[83]

mutation may get along well enough until he be subjected to some exceptional test; but an external agent, such as an injury, of a degree harmless to an ordinary individual, may have serious consequences for him.

Unfavourable mutations of minor kinds may cause disfigurement or may inconvenience their subjects in a variety of ways, but may nevertheless recur in successive generations of a family. The conditions of civilized life tend to favour the survival of such defects; a brain worker may be little handicapped by a structural deformity of a minor kind. More serious departures from the normal may greatly diminish the chance of the sufferer's survival into adult life, and tend to die out. Others again, such as the more extreme kinds of cardiac malformations, are incompatible with survival.

Whilst a necessary factor in the improvement of the race through natural selection is the transmission by inheritance of such favourable mutations as may occur, there is abundant evidence of the hereditary transmission of such unfavourable mutations as those which entail unusual liability to disease.

IV

INHERITANCE OF MORBID LIABILITIES*

Patrius hic illi, nam plerumque morbi quoque, per successiones quasdam, ut alia traduntur.—PLINY THE YOUNGER. c. A.D. 96.

IT is obvious that the importance of heredity, in connexion with the inborn factors in disease, can hardly be exaggerated, nor can it be doubted that, apart from

---

* *Section IV* In this section, Garrod is at pains to sort out transmission by heredity from other kinds. The treatment at this distance seems obvious, but a patronizing view of so rudimentary a description is seen to be unjust when we realize that, while he was writing this book, others, particularly in America, were describing the supposed Mendelian origins of poverty, criminality, and fecklessness.

direct infection of one member by another, or very special conditions of environment, a malady which occurs in several generations of a family with more than average frequency, does so in virtue of some inborn peculiarity of the stock.

Some of the chief difficulties which, until recent times, surrounded the study of inheritance have now been overcome, thanks to the work of Francis Galton and Gregor Mendel, and those who have carried on so assiduously the researches which they initiated.

Such problems as that of atavism and the skipping of generations, and the 'knight's move' inheritance of haemophilia and colour blindness, have lost most of their obscurity, and no longer present any great difficulty of interpretation.

It is not possible, in such an essay as this, to attempt to give any general account of the modern views on heredity, and it will be necessary, whilst speaking of their bearing upon the particular problems here discussed, to assume that the reader has at least some acquaintance with the Mendelian theory and the views of Galton.

It must be recognized, at the outset, that a disease or anomaly which is present at birth is not necessarily inborn. There are some diseases which may be acquired *in utero*, such as congenital syphilis, and some congenital deformities are the results of intra-uterine amputations or minor injuries. Obviously all such may be excluded from this inquiry.

The once widespread tradition of the very hereditary nature of tuberculosis, dates from the days before the infective origin of that disease was recognized, and when it was a common occurrence for brothers and sisters to succumb, one after another, to tuberculosis caught by one from another. The adoption of precautions against infection, such as destruction of sputum, improved ventilation, instead of rigid exclusion of fresh air, and the encouragement of outdoor life, have greatly diminished the frequency of such occurrences, and have diminished the importance of the part assigned to heredity in connexion with tuberculous affections.

On the other hand, the investigations of Karl Pearson,[1] Stocks,[2] and Govearts,[3] who employed statistical methods, and dealt with thousands of cases, revealed a somewhat higher incidence of tuberculosis in members of families in which the disease has occurred in previous generations than in those in which no such family history is forthcoming.

It must be borne in mind that the occurrence of the same malady, and especially of a common malady, in several members of a family, may be fortuitous, and it is essential to employ the method of control when estimating the value of evidence of inherited liability which such occurrences supply. We need to know not

[1] Drapers' Company Research Memoirs: *Studies in Natural Deterioration*, No. II, 1905.
[2] *Ann. Eugenics*, 1927, ii. 41; and 1928, ii. 84.
[3] *Eugenics Rev.*, 1926–7, xvii. 12.

only the proportion of subjects of the disease in whose families it has previously occurred, but also the proportion of unaffected individuals with such family histories, and the frequency of such histories in members of the community at large.

It is equally important that the influence of heredity shall not be under-estimated, as it well may be, seeing that the inheritance of a particular malady may be masked, and a Mendelian recessive quality may remain latent through several generations—the atavism of the older physicians. When such intervals occur the history of previous occurrence of the malady may only be elicited by diligent inquiry,* if at all, for few of us are able to give any account of the ailments of our great-grandparents.

It should be noted, too, that experience shows that when tabulating recorded cases of a malady, the absence from the records of any mention of its occurrences in past generations, or of consanguinity of parents, cannot be taken as evidence of there having been none such.

Some peculiarity of environment is among possible causes of the family occurrence of maladies, but is little likely to lead to error. A deleterious trade carried on by successive generations, such as steel grinding, or contamination of the water-supply with lead, are cases in point. In the case of such diseases as goitre, endemic in particular regions, the members of the community and not of particular families are likely to be affected.

Mendelian studies throw very valuable light upon morbid predispositions, and numbers of human anoma-

* *diligent inquiry* How many doctors engage in a 'diligent inquiry' when taking a family history? How many try to elicit evidence of consanguinity?

[87]

lies are mutations which are either Mendelian dominants or recessives. But, since for obvious reasons the relative numbers of normal and abnormal offspring in the small human families supply little information as compared with the results of experimental breeding of prolific animals, it is mainly by the application to man of the results obtained by such experimental breeding that progress has been made.

An only child may be merely the firstborn of a family, and miscarriages would need to be taken into account in reckoning human families, and at the best the figures dealt with would be incomparably smaller than those relating to mice or rabbits, and still more to such an insect as drosophila.

Albinism,* a mutation occurring alike in man and lower animals, is clearly shown by experimental breeding to be a Mendelian recessive mutation, such as can only appear when both parents, although they may themselves be normally pigmented, contribute recessive gametes. If both parents be albinos all their offspring will be albinos. So long as one parent is a *true* dominant, normally pigmented, and contributes *only* dominant gametes, none of the children will be albinos; but, on the other hand, one parent or both parents may appear to be normal and yet produce both dominant and recessive gametes. Albinos may appear amongst the children of such parents, but several albino-free generations may elapse before a mating again occurs between parents who both produce recessive gametes.

* *Albinism*   A topic in Garrod's *Croonian lectures* and in both editions of *Inborn errors of metabolism.*

[88]

As William Bateson[1] was the first to point out, such a mating is far more likely to occur when a member of an albinotic family marries a cousin, also a member of that family, than when he or she marries into a different family, especially if the recessive characteristic be a rare one. The rarer the anomaly the higher should be the proportion of its subjects whose parents are consanguineous.

Hence it comes about that albinism, which is a rare anomaly, and has been shown to be recessive, is met with, with quite unusual frequency, in the children of consanguineous*marriages. Whereas marriages of first cousins number from one to eight per cent. of all marriages in this country, the percentage of first-cousin marriages amongst parents of albinos is about forty per cent.

In estimating such percentages a sibship containing several albino brothers and sisters should be taken as the unit, not the individual albino. The number of marriages which result in albino offspring, and not the number of albinos whose parents are consanguineous is in question.

It should be noted that the marriage of cousins as such does not favour the occurrence of such anomalies, but the union of cousins both of whom are members of the family in which the anomaly runs, and both of whom contribute recessive gametes.

It is obvious that we are justified in arguing that an

[1] *Report of the Evolution Committee of the Royal Society*, 1902, No. 1, p. 133, note.

3482   I

* *consanguineous* Whereas rare autosomal alleles are more likely to be associated with homozygous expression when the consanguinity rate is high, the more prevalent autosomal recessive phenotypes are likely to exhibit increased rates of consanguinity.

anomaly which cannot be made the subject of experimental breeding in lower animals is a recessive character, if, like albinism,* it is wont to appear in several children of parents who are apparently normal, and if a large proportion of its subjects are children of consanguineous unions. Alcaptonuria† is an example of such anomalies. It is not known to occur in lower animals, but in its incidence the above conditions are exactly fulfilled.

Of special interest to clinical workers and to students of heredity alike, are the maladies which behave as what are known as sex-linked recessives. Of such haemophilia offers a most striking example, as also does pseudo-hypertrophic muscular dystrophy, both of which are transmitted by normal females to their male offspring. It might be supposed that since few of the sufferers marry or beget children, that fact might be an important factor in determining this type of inheritance; but such explanation is excluded by the fact that the practically innocuous colour blindness is handed down in the same manner. The Mendelian explanation of such sex-linked transmission and the part played therein by the so-called X chromosome will be found in the writings which deal with that subject.

There are other anomalies which behave as dominant characters, occur in parents and children, and in a large proportion of the offspring of those who exhibit them. Of such polydactyly affords a striking example, and of family diseases haemolytic jaundice.

* *albinism*   Albinism was among the first diseases illustrating genetic heterogeneity in a particular Mendelian phenotype. Trevor-Roper (1952) described non-albino offspring of biological parents who were themselves albino. This unorthodox event is explained by recessive alleles at two different loci, one set causing the albinism in the mother, the other in the father. Offspring can only be double heterozygotes, never homozygotes for the albino phenotype(s).

If we attempt to apply Bateson's law of 'presence and absence' to human abnormalities difficulties are apt to be encountered. Whereas some recessive anomalies appear to be due to absence of some factor, a ferment in some cases, and excess of digits is obviously dominant, as Bateson's law requires, brachydactyly, with deficient number of phalanges, also behaves as a dominant. It is probable that in some at least of the apparently paradoxical instances more than one factor is concerned.

In recent years a considerable amount of information bearing upon the inheritance of human anomalies and liabilities to disease has been accumulated. In a recent work Ruggles Gates[1]*has brought together and discussed the material already available, and supplies a copious bibliography of the subject. To this and other books by British and Continental writers, the reader is referred for further information, which is outside the scope of this essay. O. Naegeli's[2] suggestive monograph may be mentioned specially.

To some examples of morbid heredity, which are of chief importance in illustration of questions here dealt with, it will be necessary to refer in later chapters.

In Francis Galton's fascinating book, entitled *Enquiries into Human Faculty*, there is a chapter upon the histories of twins, in which he remarks that 'the steady and pitiless march of the hidden weaknesses of our

[1] *Heredity in Man*, 1929.
[2] *Allgemeine Konstitutionslehre*, 1927.

† *alcaptonuria* Another topic in Garrod's *Croonian lectures* and in both editions of *Inborn errors of metabolism*.

* *Ruggles Gates* His book was a precursor to McKusick's *Mendelian inheritance in man*. There were three editions; the third published in 1946 appeared in two volumes. There were several hundred entries, but the material was neither collected nor listed in any systematic way.

constitutions, through illness to death, is painfully revealed by these histories of twins'.

The subject is closely allied to that of heredity, if not actually a part thereof.

No other two human beings are so much alike as are twins developed from a single ovum. Their likenesses of outward form are proverbial, and have supplied the plots of tales and dramas. That such twins also resemble each other in mental attributes, disposition, and tastes, is equally well recognized; and it may safely be inferred that the resemblances extend still deeper, to their tissue structure, and to the metabolic processes which constitute their chemical life. It has been shown that there are close resemblances of such essentially individual features as finger prints, sole prints, and blood groups.

Here obviously is a most promising field for inquiry into the inborn factors in disease, for, as His says[1], when there occur in uniovular twins, at like ages and with similar courses, diseases, such as pneumonia or rheumatism, which we are accustomed to regard as maladies due to exposure or occupation, we recognize the powerful influence of constitution upon them.

A large amount of information upon this subject is available, but much of it has not the accuracy demanded, if the evidence is to be regarded as conclusive. What is needed[*] is a collective investigation based upon information supplied by medical men who have been in contact with the twins from birth upwards,

[1] *Ueber die natürliche Ungleichheit der Menschen,* 1928, p. 18.

[*] *What is needed* At a time when most of the medical literature consisted of observations that we might today call anecdotal, Garrod insisted upon, and in his own work employed, careful quantitative analysis.

supplemented by other information from lying-in wards and hospital notes. In Galton's chapter, based upon answers to a questionnaire, the information was for the most part supplied by the twins or their parents, and little of it by their medical attendants.

On the other hand, notable contributions from the medical side have been made by George Murray[1] and E. A. Cockayne[2] in this country, and by Siemens[3] and others in Germany. Julius Bauer,[4] in his book on Constitution, cites a number of examples of disease in twins in his discussion of constitutional factors in particular diseases.

Obviously it is essential that in any collective investigation of the subject the inquiries must discriminate between true, uniovular twins and those developed from separate ova, but the latter will be of use as controls. In so discriminating it is easy enough to discard all cases in which the twins are of different sexes, as being obviously binovular, but it is far from easy to discriminate between mono- and hetero-zygotic twins of the same sex, and the latter, according to Newman, constitute half of the total number of twins of one sex. Evidence of a single placenta, of one chorionic and two amniotic membranes is essential when dealing with crucial cases. Apart from such cases the error resulting from accept-

[1] *Lancet,* 1925, i. 529.

[2] *Brit. J. Child. Dis.,* 1911, viii. 487.

[3] *Zwillingspathologie.* 1924.

[4] *Die konstitutionelle Disposition zu inneren Krankheiten,* 2nd ed. 1921.

ance as presumably uniovular of twins of the same sex, and whose likeness to each other is conspicuously greater than that of ordinary brothers or sisters, will not be a large one. As examples of the crucial questions referred to, in which such evidence does not suffice, may be quoted that of differences of blood groups in twins, and the occurrence of Mongolian idiocy in one of the pair.

The number of records which fulfil the strict requirements are very small, but the following may be quoted as such. Cockayne and Sheldon[1] described the cases of male twins both of whom exhibited signs of congenital pyloric stenosis in the earliest months of life. In both cases the diagnosis was confirmed at an operation. It was testified by the midwife who attended the mother that there had been one placenta, one chorion, and two amniotic sacs.

Other cases of pyloric stenosis in identical twins have been recorded.

There is much evidence which hardly admits of question, of the tendency of the so-called identical twins to develop along similar lines, even when their surroundings and upbringing are different. In Galton's[2] words, 'they continue their lives, keeping time like two watches, hardly to be thrown out of accord, except by some physical jar'.

There is also an impressive mass of evidence that

[1] *Proc. Roy. Soc. Med.*, 1928, xxi. 1260.
[2] *Inquiries into Human Faculty*, 1883, p. 235.

[94]

true twins are wont to suffer from the same illnesses almost simultaneously, even though living far apart and in different circumstances.

One is tempted to be sceptical as to such records, but it is hard to doubt the testimony of Trousseau[1] as regards the often quoted case of twin brothers who were attacked simultaneously with 'rheumatic ophthalmia', in Paris and Vienna respectively, and who both suffered from asthma. In this, as in other recorded cases the one twin foretold the other's attack. Trousseau adds, that however singular this story may appear, the fact is none the less exact; it was not told him by others, but he has seen it himself; and has seen other similar cases in his practice.

There are not a few instances of similar troubles developed by twins well on in life, and in some of these the maladies observed have not been such as might be expected to be hereditary.

Among such are Hodgkin's disease, lymphatic leukaemia, Hirschsprung's disease, and Hanot's cirrhosis of the liver, papilloma of the larynx, and even empyema and pneumonia. Amongst the records scattered through Bauer's book are some of Fröhlich's syndrome, calcaruria, renal tuberculosis, and various nervous disorders, including myatonia congenita and spastic paraplegia. Such cases are not numerous enough to serve as bases of generalization, but they emphasize the desirability of systematic research upon rigid lines.

[1] *Clinique Médicale*, 1861, tome i, p. 523.

Of exceptional interest and importance are the examples of diabetes in twins collected by W. Stanley Curtis [1] of Boston. They relate to thirteen pairs of twins, several of which were under observation in the Joslin clinic, and it is necessary in this connexion to take into account not only the several kinds of twinship but also the several kinds of glycosuria, some of which appear to be manifestations of definitely inborn peculiarities, such as the glycosuria without hyperglycaemia, the so-called diabetes innocens.

Of Curtis's thirteen pairs of twins one pair was of different sexes, and two other pairs are described as not homologous, although of the same sex. The remainder are classed as identical twins. It is of interest to note that the ages at the period of onset of the diabetes varied within such wide limits as three to sixty years. Twin brothers of fifty-nine, died of diabetes within two months of each other, and brothers of sixty within a few weeks. Yet a third pair of brothers succumbed to the disease within four months of each other, at the age of twenty-seven.

Such cases recall Galton's simile of the watches which run down together.

In other cases there were long intervals between the onsets of the malady; and as evidence of the difficulties which beset such inquiries, Curtis tells that the mother of the twins of different sexes declared that they always had the same diseases.

[1] *Jour. Amer. Med. Ass.*, 1929, xcii. 952.

[96]

It must be acknowledged that there is something uncanny about the diseases of twins.

Each of the subjects so far discussed has important bearings upon questions of constitution, of human individuality, and upon what Langdon Brown[1] has called predestination to disease. The attempt may now be made to apply the knowledge gained in recent years of the chemical constitution and activities of the human body to the elucidation of the processes at work in rendering it unduly liable to, or unduly immune from, diseases of various kinds.

[1] *Brit. Med. Jour.*, 1930, i. 525.

PART II

THE SEVERAL KINDS OF PRE-
DISPOSITION

V

STRUCTURE AND FORM IN RELATION
TO DISEASE

*Each patient has a pathological, as well as a mental and social individu-
ality.*—THOMAS LAYCOCK, 1862.

THE relationship of structure to disease has to be
considered under two main aspects. In the first
place peculiarities of form or feature may serve as labels
indicative of liability to particular maladies, although no
obvious part in the causation of those maladies can be
assigned to them. On the other hand, some deviations
from the average build and structure of the species
render their possessors liable to pathological accidents
of various kinds.

It has long been recognized that, as regards their
liability to disease, people fall into different classes, and
that such liabilities may be associated with differences
of structure and feature; so that the several 'temperaments', to use the term in its older sense, may often be
recognized by mere inspection.

Various factors doubtless contribute to the production of those groups of individuals who resemble each
other, not only in outward form, but also in physiological

[98]

and mental processes. Amongst these the accumulated effects of inheritance play important parts.

In a race such as ours, which results from the fusion of a number of strains, and especially of Kelt, Anglo-Saxon, and Northman, racial peculiarities must contribute largely; and just as racial characteristics extend to the forms and agglutinations of the red corpuscles of the blood, so also there is a considerable mass of evidence pointing to racial liabilities to, and immunity from particular diseases.*

In recent years the study of such individual differences of structure, and of the morbid proclivities associated with them, has been approached along modern scientific lines, and by the employment of anthropometric methods. Such anthropometric studies, together with others involving different methods, but similar in their aims, are being pursued in the 'Constitutional Clinics' which have been established in several centres. George Draper,[1] who presides over such a clinic in New York, has already published a volume dealing with what he describes as the 'anatomical panel', and which embodies the results of large numbers of measurements, and deals with statistics relating to many individual men and women as regards their stature, girth, weight, and any physical peculiarities of feature or limb which they exhibit. This investigation is only a part of that contemplated in Draper's scheme, which embraces also physiological, psychological, and immunological panels.

[1] *Human Constitution*, 1924.

* *racial liabilities . . . and immunity* Population genetics explains how genes have segregated historically in populations. Genetic epidemiology is concerned with the genetics of contemporary populations and how genes predispose to disease. If genetic epidemiology is a 'modern' discipline Garrod is one of its intellectual founders.

In his anatomical studies Draper applies the yard-stick to the outward manifestations of the various 'temperaments' upon which earlier physicians laid so much stress, and from the data so obtained he claims to be able to distinguish types of individuals who are liable to suffer from particular kinds of disease, such as chole-lithiasis, duodenal ulceration, and pernicious anaemia.

In the production of those structural characteristics which we speak of as family likenesses and racial resemblances, and in so doing bear witness to their hereditary transmission, a large share must be assigned to the endocrine glands, those balanced regulators which, in virtue of the hormones which they secrete, exercise control over the metabolic processes, and through these over the bodily functions, and play most important parts in determining the dimensions and contours of the body. Indeed Pende[1] of Turin, who is director of the Constitutional Clinic in that city, would assign to these glands the leading role in determining the constitution of a man.

In so far as the various factors concerned in the making of a human individuality are to a large extent interdependent, it may be expected that the more obvious peculiarities, those of structure and form, will serve as outward and visible signs of other and more subtle differences, such as predisposition to diseases, and even of a primary peculiarity of chemical structure and form, upon which all others depend.

[1] *Constitutional Inadequacies,* 1928.

To turn to the second division of the subject under discussion, namely the part played by anatomical anomalies in predisposing their subjects to disease, it is surprising, at first sight, to find how small that part is. Important as is the part which disease plays as an instrument of natural selection, it is rather those who are functionally than physically unfit who are weeded out by its means.

Yet in extreme cases congenital malformations may be incompatible with survival; or as is the case with certain cardiac defects, may seriously curtail life. Malformations of less degree may place their subjects at serious disadvantage, by disfiguring them, by hindering them in earning a living, or by impairing their powers of self defence.

It is hardly necessary to point out that malformations differ widely in kind. Some are due to failure to complete some structure, and to this class of malformations by defect belong hare-lip, cleft-palate, and spina bifida. Others are malformations by excess, such as extra digits, and others again, such as branchial clefts, present persistent vestigial remnants. Many malformations are obviously heritable, either as dominant or recessive characteristics, and it would seem that in some families what is inherited is a tendency to structural variations, rather than any individual anomaly.

On the other hand, it cannot be supposed that the evolution of the human frame has reached its limits, nor that all variations of form are necessarily harmful;

although in the course of ages the body has become so well adapted to its surroundings that, in its ordinary environment, any conspicuous change is more likely to be harmful than beneficial.

When an important organ is malformed its function may be impaired. The subjects of congenital cystic disease of the kidneys[*] may show few symptoms for years, but eventually they usually succumb to progressive renal disease. That this anomaly is inborn is shown by its occurrence in successive generations of a family; as in families described by H. W. B. Cairns[1] and C. J. Fuller,[2] in one of which it was traced through four generations. There is still much to be learned as to the initial stages of the anomaly, and some hesitation is permissible in deciding whether to place it under the heading of malformations or that of tissue-defects. The cyanosis and clubbing of the digits in cases of cardiac malformation may be cited as other examples of secondary effects of structural anomalies.

In a case seen by the writer, a young woman died suddenly in an uraemic convulsion, due to pressure of an enlarging uterus upon a single small kidney, situated in the hollow of the sacrum; again abnormal mesenteries of the caecum or colon may lead to intussusception or volvulus, even in later life.

Occasionally a definite clinical picture is presented by a group of congenital anomalies, and examples there-

[1] *Quart. Jour. Med.*, 1924–5, xviii. 359.
[2] Ibid., 1928–9, xxii. 567.

* *congenital cystic disease of the kidneys* A polymorphic marker has been found on chromosome 16 for dominantly inherited adult-onset polycystic kidney disease (Reeders *et al.* 1985). The form of 'cystic disease' Garrod had in mind appears to be autosomal dominant.

of may be met with from time to time. For example, an almost complete absence of the muscles of the abdominal [1] wall occurs in association with enormous dilatation of the ureters, and of the bladder which is usually attached to the umbilicus. The condition is usually fatal in infancy, but some subjects have survived to adult life. It is not certain which is the primary event, but examination of subjects of the anomalies leaves little room for doubt that the abdominal distension due to the huge bladder leads to atrophy of the affected muscles.

However, such combinations and happenings rank rather as clinical curiosities than as examples of structural predisposition to morbid states; and as such they contribute but little to the elucidation of the problems of predisposition. Far more germane thereto, but still of the nature of curiosities, are the cases in which a malformed part serves as a seat of election of an infective process. Thus it is a recognized fact that malformed cardiac valves are favourite seats of malignant endocarditis, and specimens are to be seen in museums in which the abnormal curtains alone have been attacked. Yet such cases also contribute only a very minute fraction to the total of cases of such endocarditis.

Vestigial remnants, also, may be sources of danger to those who possess them. Thus a Meckel's diverticulum may not only give rise to strangulation of the intestine, or to intussusception, but it also appears to

[1] Garrod, A. E. and Davies, Ll. W., *Med.-Chir. Trans.*, 1905, lxxxviii. 363.

be specially liable to become the seat of inflammation or ulceration of the peptic type, and the presence of gastric mucous membrane in such diverticula has been described by M. J. Stewart.[1] It may even be suggested that the vermiform appendix is become increasingly ill-adapted to the conditions of modern civilization, and that its increasing liability to inflammation is more than apparent.

The phthinoid chest-forms, upon which so much stress used to be laid, may have owed their evil reputations to their being ill-adapted for thorough ventilation of the lungs, and especially of their apices, and so offering favourable opportunities for the lodgment of tubercle bacilli.

Hurst's[2] observations on differences in the forms of stomachs, and the pathological events dependent thereupon, are of special interest in relation to the subject under discussion.

X-ray examinations of numbers of normal and abnormal individuals have convinced him that the conditions which have been described as gastric hypertonus and gastroptosis respectively are dependent upon the form of the stomach, and not upon its tone; that a stomach formerly said to be in a condition of hypertonus is in reality a short stomach, and that gastroptosis is the

[1] Hurst, A. F., and Stewart, M. J., *Gastric and Duodenal Ulcer*, 1929, p. 77.
[2] 'The Constitutional Factor in Disease', *Brit. Med. Jour.*, 1927, i. 823.

sign of a long one. Both may be regarded as variants from the average form of stomach met with in normal people, as being independent of gastric tone, and of the amount of support afforded by the abdominal wall.

Moreover, hyperchlorhydria, which has been shown by Ryle [1] and others to be commonly associated with a short stomach, and hypochlorhydria usually associated with a long one, are physiological variations from the average of gastric secretion. They are both met with in normal individuals. It is not suggested that the type of secretion is *dependent* upon the length of the stomach, but that the associated conditions are wont to coexist in individuals of particular structure and build. Furthermore, such conditions may predispose to disease of particular kinds; such as duodenal ulcer, which is apt to occur in those whose stomachs are short, and whose gastric juice is unduly rich in hydrochloric acid.

The intimate connexion between structure and function here suggested, has been alluded to in earlier chapters. The trifling deviations of form and function which are revealed by anthropometry, and by physiological tests may be looked upon as slight oscillations, such as are bound to occur, to one side or another of an imaginary normal line. Such trifling innovations may furnish clues to the gifted facial diagnostician, and wider deviations may offer much more obvious warning signals, even though the anomaly may be one of function and not of structure.

[1] *Guy's Hosp. Gaz.*, 1926, xl. 546.

3482   I.

VI

TISSUE DEFECTS.—ABIOTROPHIES

*Es angeborene embryonale Defekte gibt, bei deren Bestehen die normale
Funktion schon eine Schädigung bedeute.*—O. ROSENBACH. 1891.

IN the conditions next to be discussed, the congenital
defects are not of particular organs, but of tissues of
particular kinds. In some instances there are present
from birth, obvious changes in the affected tissues, inherited from former generations, and which have none
of the characters of progressive diseases. Sometimes the
only outward sign of defect of internal tissues is some
warning signal, in a conspicuous situation, such as blueness of the sclerotics of the eyes. In some instances
there develops upon the top of the congenital defect a
progressive morbid process, and, occasionally, stationary
tissue defects and progressive changes are mixed together to form a complex clinical picture. Lastly, there
are maladies, inherited and obviously inborn, in which
there are no obvious tissue defects at birth, nor in early
childhood, but in which there appear, at some period
in early life, signs of a progressive disease. The best
examples of these last are to be found in the heredo-
familial diseases of the neuro-muscular system, to which
Gowers gave the name of 'abiotrophies'.*

Such conditions found no place in the diathetic lists
of our forefathers, although they offer some of the most
striking examples of inborn tendencies to special forms
of disease, or more strictly, to disease of special tissues.

* 'Abiotrophies' Abiotrophy is a word that vanished from medical texts
in the 1930s. It means a loss of the cells of particular tissues. The diseases are
now classified under the headings of organs, e.g. skin, muscle, or central
nervous system. Most of the conditions Garrod mentions are now recognized
to be monogenic in origin. McKusick (1983) lists many 'abiotrophies'.

Doubtless their omission was mainly due to the fact that very little was known about these maladies at the time when the idea of diatheses was to the fore, and that of some of them nothing was then known. They have no place in Hutchinson's *Pedigree of Disease*, although its author mentions that he has met, in his practice, with inherited liability of kindred tissues to exhibit inflammation of peculiar forms, at certain ages, and as effects of very insignificant causes.

Among the tissue defects which may be regarded as congenital malformations rather than as progressive maladies, those which involve the surface tissues are naturally the most obvious. They are usually hereditary in a pronounced degree. Ichthyosis, and tilosis of the palms and soles are familiar examples, but in recent years increasing attention has been given to a rare and most remarkable form of ectodermal defect. It has been described as incomplete development of the epidermis and its dependencies, amounting sometimes to its absence over circumscribed areas. The anomaly was first described by Goeckermann[1] in the year 1920, and among those who have studied it since may be mentioned Christ,[2] MacKee and Andrews,[3] and Falkoner[4] of Capetown.

One of its most striking features is a partial or com-

---

[1] *Arch. Dermat. and Syph.*, 1920, i. 396.
[2] *Arch. f. Dermat. u. Syph.*, 1913, cxvi. 685.
[3] *Arch. Dermat. and Syph.*, 1924, x. 673.
[4] *Lancet*, 1929, ii. 656.

plete absence of teeth. The nasal bridge is usually depressed, the skin is dry, smooth and glossy; and owing to the lack of sweat glands the victims of the anomaly suffer much discomfort in hot weather. The sebaceous glands are also absent and the hairs scanty.

The defect is strongly hereditary and in some instances the dental defect has been the only visible sign in some members of an affected family.

Here we have an example of a heritable defect limited to tissues of a particular class, namely ectodermal, which are embryologically connected.

In another group it is in the bony structures that the shortcomings are mostly observed. A noteworthy example is afforded by the hereditary form of brittleness of the bones which has been observed in large numbers of the members of successive generations of some affected families. The fragility is apparently due to a defect of the mesenchyme, leading to an imperfect formation of connective tissues, rather than to any imperfect laying down of calcium salts in the bones; for the blue colour of the sclerotics of the eyes of those members of a family in which the condition occurs, is certainly due to imperfection of the fibrous tissue of the sclerotics, which, being less opaque than it should be, allows the black pigment of the choroid to show through it. An analogous blue colour, due to the blackened cartilage showing through the skin, is seen in the hollows of the ears in cases of ochronosis.

The blue sclerotics[*] serve as warning signals of the

* *blue sclerotics* A sign of osteogenesis imperfecta but only in some of its forms. Mutations at the collagen loci on chromosomes 7 and 17 (and elsewhere) affect the composition of the collagen and the stability of the fibril (Byers and Benadio 1985). Different mutations affect collagen in different ways and confer different phenotypes.

presence of the anomaly of the bones, and also bear eloquent witness to the inborn and congenital nature of that anomaly.

The affected members of such a family suffer repeated fractures of bones from what appear to be wholly inadequate causes; their skeletons are unable to bear the wear and tear of daily life.

The fractures occur at any period of life, from early childhood onwards; and as life goes on the majority of the victims develop the changes in the aural structures known as otosclerosis, manifested by progressive deafness. There can be no question of the association, for otosclerosis has been met with in many subjects and in members of various affected families.

Here then we have a very instructive combination of three factors in a morbid picture. First the visible warning signal the blueness of the sclerotics, secondly the inability to resist slight traumata, manifested in the repeated fractures of bones as the results of slight injuries, and thirdly the progressive deterioration of the structures of the ears, the otosclerosis. And with it all we have one of the most striking of known examples of hereditary transmission of a defect met with in the whole field of pathology.

In recent years the use of the X-rays has brought to light a still rarer form of brittleness of bones. In cases of this condition the shadows cast by the bones are uniformly dark, as if they were solid throughout, which they actually are in advanced cases. Here the brittle-

ness is presumably due to loss of tubular structure, and
also to diminished elasticity of the affected bones. It
would seem that such osteosclerosis[*] is progressive, for
various degrees of obliteration of the marrow cavities
have been observed; but it is so rare, and has been so
seldom met with, that it would be premature to base any
sweeping conclusions upon the scanty knowledge which
we have of it. It is almost certainly a Mendelian recessive, and like other such, has been met with unduly
often in children of first cousins. It is a matter of no
small interest that in some advanced cases of such osteosclerosis, there has been enlargement of the spleen and
lymphatic glands, as if to compensate for the destruction of the bone-marrow.

That remarkable and bizarre malady known as
myositis ossificans progressiva is of even greater interest
in connexion with our subject. In it also the mesenchyme
is the seat of the defect, and Julius Bauer suggests that
in those who suffer from it the cells of the mesenchyme
retain the power which they normally lose, of forming
bony tissue [1]; for it is in the connective tissue around the
affected muscles that the osseous deposits are formed.
It is noteworthy that a similar bone-formation is occasionally seen as a localized result of a severe local injury.

It must be acknowledged that the evidence of inheritance of myositis ossificans is, up to now, very scanty,
and in the majority of cases in which inquiry upon this

[1] *Die konstitutionelle Disposition zu inneren Krankheiten*, 2nd ed.,
1921, p. 330.

[*] *osteosclerosis* Garrod is referring apparently to osteopetrosis of which
there are several Mendelian forms. A newly recognized recessive form is
associated with a mutation on chromosome 8 causing deficiency of carbonic
anhydrase-II (Sly *et al.* 1985).

point has been made, no evidence of family occurrence has been forthcoming. This fact presents a serious obstacle to the inclusion of the disease in the group under discussion. Against it may be set the remarkable fact that in no less than 70 per cent. of all recorded cases there have been congenital deformities of the great toes, and in some cases, of the thumbs also. The nature of the deformities is not so constant as their seats, but in most instances the affected digits are shortened, either by suppression of a phalanx or by fusion of phalanges.

In one instance a father who had such digital defor-mities, but no myositis, begat a son with identical de-formities who developed myositis ossificans in early childhood.

It is difficult to imagine what is the connecting link between the malformations and the malady, unless the latter has an inborn basis, and as has been mentioned in connexion with ectodermal defect, the widening of the extent of a tissue anomaly in successive generations of a family is not an uncommon phenomenon.

We are probably justified in including amongst tissue defects certain familial and hereditary diseases which are characterized by anomalies of the red blood cor-puscles* and leucocytes, and especially that known as acholuric jaundice, or, preferably, as congenital haemo-lytic jaundice. It was Chauffard who first pointed out that the red corpuscles of the subjects of that malady undergo haemolysis in saline solutions not sufficiently dilute to haemolyse those of normal blood, or as it is

* *red corpuscles* The disease is apparently congenital spherocytosis which is associated with a defect in the protein, spectrin; the gene for spectrin maps to chromosome 14. There are other Mendelian disorders of erythrocyte structure (Lux 1983).

usually stated, are abnormally 'brittle'. Naegeli[1] made the further observation that the red corpuscles of a patient with haemolytic jaundice, although they appear unduly small under the microscope, actually exceed normal erythrocytes in volume. From this he concludes that they are more globular in form.

The peculiarities of the red corpuscles, their brittleness and unusual form, are obviously independent of the medium in which they are suspended, and it has not, apparently, been shown that normal red corpuscles are rendered brittle by contact with the serum of a subject of haemolytic jaundice.

Naegeli holds, moreover, that the abnormality of the corpuscles is the primary feature of the malady which only manifests itself by visible signs under the influence of external agencies such as infections or poisons. The enlargement of the spleen and the haemolysis he regards as secondary phenomena, for he finds that the abnormal form of the erythrocytes persists, and their brittleness is only diminished slightly after removal of the spleen. The remarkable improvement which follows splenectomy, and which amounts, in some cases, to practical recovery, he attributes to the withdrawal of the haemolytic action of the spleen. Lastly, Naegeli classes the condition as a mutation of the Mendelian dominant class.

Hawkins and Dudgeon[2] made the interesting sugges-

[1] *Allgemeine Konstitutionslehre*, 1927.
[2] *Quarterly Journal of Medicine*, 1908–9, ii. 165.

tion that the brittleness of the red corpuscles may be due to a deficient stability of the haemoglobin contained in them; interesting because if verified it would bring congenital haemolytic jaundice into line with morbid states obviously due to chemical abnormalities.

Yet another borderland malady, on the frontier of structural and chemical anomalies, is that which is called, after its discoverer, Gaucher's disease.* Here, as in the instance of dystrophia myotonica, to be referred to later, we meet with a history of greater and greater extension of a clinical and pathological picture, each step forward throwing fresh light upon the pathogeny of the trouble. The story dates back to the year 1882, in which Gaucher [1] described a condition of primary epithelioma of the spleen, a kind of splenomegaly met with by him in a child, and characterized by the presence in the splenic tissue of many large hyaline cells which stained only feebly. Since then a number of such cases have been observed, in all of which there has been the same microscopic picture, which is quite unlike any observed in other varieties of splenic disease. As the fresh cases were investigated it soon became evident that this was no variety of malignant tumour, and that the morbid changes were by no means limited to the spleen.

As the disease progresses the liver undergoes great enlargement also, and the haemopoietic tissues generally, including the bone marrow, become involved, and not merely in a secondary manner; for the characteristic

---

[1] *De l'Épithélioma Primitif de la Rate. Thèse de Paris*, 1882.

3482   M

* *Gaucher's disease* Another Mendelian disease, in fact, an inborn error of metabolism deriving from deficiency of glucocerebrosidase; it occurs in several forms (Brady and Barranger 1983). The gene is on chromosome 1q.

hyaline Gaucher cells are found in all the affected tissues.

It has been observed, moreover, that Gaucher's disease is wont to occur in several members of a sibship, the offspring of normal parents, which suggests the probability that it is inherited as a Mendelian recessive; but consanguinity of parents has not as yet been recorded. It is noteworthy that a large proportion of the sufferers have been females. Commencing during childhood, the malady advances at a snail's pace through decades of the victim's life. Hardly any progressive malady is so extremely chronic.

In recent years much more has been learnt about Gaucher's disease. It has been shown that the cells which are the characteristic feature of the pathological picture owe their peculiar, hyaline, swollen appearance to the presence in them of a chemical compound which is not found in ordinary splenic tissue, in quantities up to 10 per cent. of the dried spleen substance. This compound, kerasin, is allied to cerebrin which was obtained from brain substance by Thudichum, and is a member of the group of galacto-lipins. Whether the kerasin is present as such, or as a constituent of a more complex molecule, and whether it is formed in or deposited in the Gaucher's cells, has not yet been determined.

Pick,[1] who is one of the most recent investigators of the malady, takes the view that it has its origin in some

[1] *Ergebn. d. inn. Med. u. Kinderheilk.*, 1926, xxix. 519.

inborn anomaly of metabolism, by which the metabolic path is perverted rather than arrested at an intermediate stage. He compares the deposition of the Gaucher substance with the similar laying down of abnormal chemical material, such as fat out of its proper place, in the reticulo-epithelial tissues of sufferers from diabetes.

To turn now to the abiotrophies of Gowers,[1] in which there is in many instances atrophy of muscular fibres or nerve cells and fibres, which Gowers described as a wasting away of tissues, as of plants without soil, and its replacement by fibrous tissue, 'tissue weed' as he called it. But this designation as tissue weed is not altogether a happy one, for the fibrous tissue may be more aptly compared to the rubble with which a breach in a fortress wall has been repaired. It represents an attempt to mend; the best that Nature can do to make good the loss.

Some of the neuro-muscular abiotrophies, and especially that peculiar kind known as pseudo-hypertrophic muscular dystrophy, are sex-linked Mendelian recessives, transmitted almost always by normal females to their male offspring. Others behave as simple recessives and some as dominant characters.

The onset of such a malady, or rather its manifestation by obvious signs, is wont to occur at about the same age in the several affected members of a sibship (a set of brothers and sisters), but there is a tendency for the age of onset to anticipate from generation to generation. As Mott suggested, but in another connexion,

[1] *Lancet*, 1902, i. 1003.

diseases which behave in this manner tend to eliminate themselves from the stock in which they occur, by a virtuous circle so to speak; whereas sex-linked recessive characters tend to secure their own survival, seeing that the healthy members of the family transmit the defect.

Up to now little is known of the state of the affected tissues in the stage before the disease becomes apparent. The rarity of most of these tissue defects renders such inquiries difficult, but systematic examination of the children of the affected families might meet with some reward. Abnormalities of individual muscles in association with the tissue defect have been described as met with in some cases, and in others, areas of change have been found in muscles not yet obviously involved. Of less importance, save as affording evidence of structural instability, are malformations of various kinds which have been met with in such cases. Such malformations of minor degree are common enough, and comparative statistics of their occurrence in myopathic and other individuals are necessary if we are to judge the value of such evidence.

The abiotrophies of the neuro-muscular system differ conspicuously amongst themselves in their clinical features, which is not surprising seeing that the clinical pictures of nervous diseases are shaped largely by the situations of the lesions. In some of them muscular atrophy is the conspicuous manifestation, in others muscular spasm, and in others again atrophy and spasm in association. Some again, such as Friedreich's ataxia, are manifested by inco-ordination and tremor. It is noteworthy, moreover, that the various types of such affections do not appear to breed true, for different members of the group have been met with in different members of the same family.

That a neuro-muscular defect may be merely the conspicuous sign of a far wider morbid picture, is well illustrated by the growth of our knowledge of that one of them which goes by the name of dystrophia myotonica.* The story is well told in a paper by Adie and Greenfield,[1] published in 1923.

The first step was the recognition, in a special group of cases of myotonia (the condition of which Thomsen's disease is the best-known form), of the association with the muscular spasm, of muscular atrophy of somewhat unusual distribution, facial, brachial, cervical, and in some cases, peroneal. This association is named, after those who first described it, the Batten, Steinert, Curschmann syndrome. The second step was the observation that, with the above syndrome, cataract is wont to be associated, either in the patients themselves, or in members of previous generations of their families. Later still, it became evident that the dystrophy, myotonia and cataract are one and all manifestations of a still more comprehensive hereditary and familial disease, amongst the other signs of which are changes in the thyroid gland, testicular atrophy, baldness, increased secretion of sweat and tears, with cyanosis and coldness of the

[1] *Brain,* 1923, xlvi. 73.

* *dystrophia myotonica*   The gene for this disease is on chromosome 19 q. Expression of this progressive dominant phenotype is exaggerated when inherited from the mother as opposed to the father. This unusual phenomenon could have several explanations; genetic imprinting is one (Monk 1987).

extremities. This somewhat confused clinical picture has suggested to some observers that behind it is a widespread defect of endocrine glands—that it is a pluriglandular syndrome, in fact.

It is noteworthy that whereas in the cases hitherto reported the dystrophy and muscular spasm have been met only in collaterals belonging to a single generation of a family, and in them has seldom developed under the age of twenty-five years, the cataract has been traced back through four or five generations of that same family.

No one who has watched the course of the diseases here grouped together under the name of tissue defects, can doubt that inborn factors play very large parts in their causation. The development of a characteristic syndrome in member after member of a family, and often in members of successive generations; its appearance at about the same period of life in the members of a generation, and its tendency, in most instances, to anticipate from generation to generation, suffice in themselves to prove the importance of the constitutional element. Further evidence is afforded by the warning signals sometimes shown, which may attract attention even during the latent period of the malady. On the other hand, it is difficult to conceive of the steady progress of such maladies unaided by any external influences, even if we are driven to invoke as such the innumerable minimal insults which constitute the wear and tear of daily life.* It may well be true as Rendu

* *wear and tear*   Garrod's idea that these genetic disorders of long latency and late onset might be brought on by, among other influences, 'the wear and tear of daily life' is very modern. In his own time, the effects of heredity and environment were thought by many to be independent.

[118]

wrote, in an article on Gout, 'C'est d'ailleurs une loi générale que le traumatisme éveille souvent la prédisposition diathésique'.

The subject of a constitutional defect who suffers from obvious lesions when exposed to some particular external influence may have remained quite unaware of his liability until he was exposed to such influence; a subject of Raynaud's disease may exhibit no symptoms until he removes from a hot climate to a cold one. Whether it would be possible by any special care to avert a neuro-muscular abiotrophy remains unknown.

Nor can any answer yet be given to the question whether, in cases of congenital and hereditary tissue defects, the structure or make-up of the affected tissues is at fault, or whether their resistance is impaired by some unusual metabolic product present in them.* The only positive indications of abnormality are afforded by Naegeli's observations upon the red blood corpuscles in congenital haemolytic jaundice, and by some abnormalities of muscle cells in Thomsen's disease and in some dystrophies, but in the blue sclerotics associated with fragility of bones there is visible evidence of tissue deficiency present from birth.

That chemical substances exercise selective action upon particular tissue is not open to doubt, as witness the staining of cartilages by homogentisic acid and of bones by porphyrin, and the deposition of sodium urate in the cartilages of the gouty; also the symptoms of not

[1] *Dict. Encyclop. des Sci. Méd.*, 1884, x. 73.

* *the question* Garrod suggests two possibilities to explain the abiotrophies; either the tissues lack some quality of endurance and so give out in time, or some abnormal metabolite damages them. Can we now make such a distinction? We do know that there is an abnormal collagen in Marfan syndrome, but we cannot make the distinction apropos of Huntingdon disease.

a few forms of acute poisoning bear witness to selective actions. However, there is as yet no evidence of the presence in the blood or tissues of any such selective agent in any of the conditions which have been considered in this chapter, with the exception of Gaucher's disease which differs in several respects from other members of the group spoken of as abiotrophies.

If the defect be in the make-up of the tissues it is probably due to errors of chemical structure, rather than to mere morphological anomaly.

Whatever their nature, the tissue defects, or some of them at least, teach us the important lesson that maladies which only manifest their presence some years after birth, or even during adult life, may have their origins in some peculiarities of the germ plasm which may be completely latent in the earlier years of life.

VII

ERRORS OF METABOLISM

Diathetic diseases are apparently generated and sustained by an intrinsic blood-poison, resulting from some perversion of the nutritive processes of the individual.—w. h. walshe, 1855.

IN the discussion of the parts played by derangements of function as inborn factors in disease, it will be convenient to consider the subject under three headings. In the first of the three sections there will call for discussion the parts played by errors of metabolism which can be detected and studied by the methods employed

[120]

in the chemical laboratory, and this study seems to bring us into closer touch than does any other with those underlying causes which determine the liabilities of some individuals and the immunities of others.

In the second section there will be considered the evidence for and against the existence of inborn predispositions to, and defences against, particular infective maladies—subjects of which our knowledge is far less precise as yet. It is well recognized that chemical agents play very important parts as means of defence of the patients, and as weapons in the armament of the invading organisms; but as yet we have no clear knowledge of such agents as chemical compounds, and can only recognize their presence by their physiological actions, and usually by single properties which they possess, just as if we knew nothing of strychnine save its power of causing convulsions, nor of morphine save as an inducer of sleep.

Yet we may confidently expect that as time goes on, antitoxins and their congeners will be isolated as pure substances, and that their constitution will be known, just as the hormones adrenalin and thyroxin have already been isolated and synthesized.

A third chapter will be devoted to a brief survey of the bearing upon our thesis of the so-called idiosyncrasies; in virtue of which substances contained in particular foods, certain drugs and exhalations of particular animals or plants produce in some people effects wholly out of proportion to any which they bring about in

3482   N

average individuals. Such effects vary from a slight and temporary discomfort to morbid syndromes which amount to severe or even fatal illnesses. Of these latter asthma offers a most striking example.

Whatever may have been at the back of the mind of Germain Sée[1] when he wrote of predisposition as 'cet état intermédiaire qui n'est pas encore la maladie—mais qui n'est déjà plus la santé parfaite', or of Jonathan Hutchinson,[2] when he spoke of a diathesis as 'any condition of prolonged peculiarity of health, giving proclivity to definite forms of disease' their definitions are applicable in a remarkable degree to the conditions which now call for consideration.

It has been seen how, in any theory of the nature of tissue defects, there are gaps which cannot be bridged over in the present state of our knowledge. The conditions now to be considered give more encouragement to students of constitutional factors, for in some at least of them it is possible to fathom the means by which predisposition to a disease is brought about.[3]

They show how a product of metabolism, when present in the tissues from birth throughout life, may work mischief in the course of years. Such a product, although not directly harmful, may nevertheless place an individual at a disadvantage, by rendering him liable to

[1] *Leçons de Pathologie expérimentale. Généralités*, p. xiii. 1867.

[2] *The Pedigree of Disease*, 1884, p. 71.

[3] Garrod, A. E., *Inborn Errors of Metabolism*, 2nd ed., 1923 (gives many references to literature of the subject).

suffer, in some obvious way, when exposed to such external influences as infections, exposure to bright light, traumata, slight or severe, or even to the wear and tear of daily life.

The chemical agent concerned may be a product of normal metabolism formed in undue amount, or an intermediate product which escapes the further changes which it normally undergoes, or possibly an abnormal product formed owing to deflexion of a metabolic process from its normal path.

The individual*who carries such a substance in his tissues can hardly be said to suffer from any disease, and it may well be that his anomaly is harmless or even helpful to him. On the other hand, he is not in perfect health if he is rendered by it unable to adjust himself to his environment, that is to say to the influences to which a man is habitually exposed.

Seeing that no two individuals of a species, nor even uniovular twins, are exactly alike in structure and outward form, seeing also that the standard of chemical structure and chemical process is no rigid one, but represents an average, it can hardly be that in their chemistry, as in their structure, any two individuals are exactly alike. There is indeed much evidence of chemical individuality, as well as of chemical specificity.

In section ii it was pointed out also, that the structure of the molecules of proteins is capable of colossal numbers of different groupings and proportional compositions, but seeing that deviations from the metabolic

* *The individual* Disease is perceived as the result of an incongruity between one's chemical individuality and the influences to which one is exposed.

average are of necessity less obvious than variations of
form, they attract comparatively little attention. It can
hardly be doubted that the great majority of minor
chemical variations have hitherto escaped observation.

The more pronounced chemical mutations which
come under observation from time to time are clearly
hereditary, and are extremely rare for the most part.
The search for minor mutations revealed by no conspicuous appearance or by response to a widely used
test, may be compared to the proverbial search for a
needle in a haystack. Hitherto, the few recognized
chemical abnormalities have attracted attention by some
warning signal, comparable to the blue sclerotics of the
subjects of fragilitas ossium. A systematic search for
chemical mutations which show no such signs would
involve elaborate metabolic studies of large numbers
of specimens from many human beings, and the labour
so expended would usually prove vain. Even a very
limited experience of such searches* served to deter the
writer from pursuing further so discouraging a task.

In connexion with the known chemical anomalies the
factor of inheritance plays a no less important part than
with structural malformations. Most of them are recessive characters in the Mendelian sense, and this
suggests that the defects are rather negative than positive. There is some tendency to sex-linkage, seeing that
in the case of those defects of which a considerable
number of examples have been observed, the males have
been about twice as numerous as the female subjects.

* *such searches* We know today of the extensive polymorphism of human
enzymes and other proteins, as well as of the DNA itself. The search for
qualitative evidence of 'chemical mutations' is no longer 'so discouraging a
task'.

It is difficult to imagine that this male preponderance, which holds good for the rare and conspicuous inborn errors of metabolism, can apply to chemical mutations in general. We can hardly suppose that the metabolism of males is far more liable to go wrong than that of females, despite its liability to do so in certain particular ways.

Although it would seem that a product of normal metabolism, even an intermediate product which should have only a momentary existence, should be little likely to be injurious to the organism in which it is formed, some at least of the chemical mutations give rise, sooner or later, to serious troubles. But such troubles are usually, if not always, provoked by some external influence. In some instances this comes about much sooner than later, as for example in haemophilia, the sex-linked recessive anomaly, due almost certainly to the lack of some enzyme concerned in the coagulation of the blood; whereas in other conditions the morbid events may only make their appearance late in life.

The subject of an inborn error of metabolism may go through life unaware of his trouble so long as he is protected from those external influences which provoke its evil manifestations.

In the days when the diatheses held the field, little was known of such chemical abnormalities, but one of them, namely cystinuria,[*] was included by Walshe in his list of diathetic disorders, contained in a lecture delivered in 1855.[1] Wollaston, who was the pioneer in the

[1] *Med. Times and Gaz.*, 1855, xxxi. 613.

[*] *cystinuria* Another topic covered in the *Croonian Lectures*; also, one of Garrod's rare misconceptions. Cystinuria is an inborn error of membrane transport not a disorder of chemical conversion. In the former, the substrate is not chemically modified. A mechanism for the cystinuria phenotype was eventually demonstrated in 1951 (Dent and Rose 1951). The mutant transport phenotype is selective for the cationic amino acids and cystine and is expressed in kidney and intestine; several alleles cause cystinuria.

chemical investigation of calculi, described, in 1810, a previously unknown variety of urinary calculus, which consisted of a chemical compound also unknown before that date. To this he gave the name of cystic oxide, for which Berzelius substituted that of cystin. Some fifteen years later the characteristic colourless hexagonal crystals of cystin were found in urine, first by Stromeyer, and soon after independently by Prout. Not until twenty years after its discovery was the fact that cystin contains sulphur recognized. For many years urinary calculi and deposits were the only known supplies of cystin. Whence it was derived remained a secret, and to all appearance it had no place in the ordinary scheme of human metabolism.

Only at the very end of the nineteenth century was it shown that cystin might be obtained in abundance by hydrolysis of hair. This discovery, which we owe to K. A. H. Mörner, was quickly followed up, and before long cystin took its place as one of the amino-acid fractions of which the protein molecules are built up, and one of the most important of these, since it contains the bulk of the sulphur which enters into the composition of proteins.

It was Alexander Marcet, a friend and contemporary of Wollaston, who first described the occurrence of cystinuria in several members of the same family. This observation has been abundantly confirmed by subsequent observers, and in some instances the anomaly has been traced through several generations. Unlike most other anomalies of its kind, the mode of inheritance of cystinuria suggests that it is a dominant character.[*]

In 1888 it was shown, by Baumann and Udranszky, that cystinurics sometimes pass in their urine, and in the faeces also, the diamines cadaverine and putrescine, which can only have been derived from the argenin and lysin of proteins. This observation also has been abundantly confirmed, but it is noteworthy that these diamines, or either of them, are not to be detected in the excreta of a large proportion of cystinurics, and when found are usually present only intermittently. More recently lysin and argenin[†] themselves have been found and other protein fractions, notably tyrosin and leucin, in the urine of some, and only some, cystinurics.

From this it would appear that what we call cystinuria, i. e. the excretion of cystin in the urine, is only the warning sign of an anomaly of protein metabolism of far wider range, which involves varying numbers of protein fractions in different cases.

It would seem also that cystin is the first fraction to be involved, but even this is uncertain, since, in the absence of cystin, with its characteristic crystalline deposits, the presence of tyrosin or leucin, and still more of the diamines, is likely to be overlooked. Nevertheless, it will hardly be doubted by those who have investigated cases of cystinuria, that in a considerable proportion of such cases cystin is the only protein fraction which is excreted unchanged in the urine.

* *dominant character* It was not until 1955 (Harris *et al.* 1955) that the heterozygous phenotype in cystinuria was shown to be either completely recessive (normal excretion of cystine and cationic amino acids) or 'incompletely recessive' (elevated excretion).

† *lysin and argenin* Omission of the final e was Garrod's custom, also misspelling of arginine. The implication of tyrosine and leucine is probably a conflation of the renal Fanconi syndrome and cystinuria. The renal Fanconi syndrome had not yet been described in 1931.

The phenomena observed suggest that there is missing in the cystinuric an enzyme or similar agent which is concerned in the desamination of the protein fractions, and that in consequence of the lack of it the stripping off of the amino-groupings from the amino-acids of some part of the proteins of the diet is not carried out, as it usually is at an early stage of protein catabolism. It would seem, further, that in consequence of the failure of the process at that stage, the protein fractions involved escape the further destruction which they normally undergo.

As far as is yet known, the presence in the blood and tissues of the unchanged amino-acids has no effect which can be described as toxic, and it would appear that the troubles to which cystinurics are exposed are wholly due to the insolubility of cystin and its consequent deposition, in crystalline form, in undesirable situations. Obviously a compound so insoluble in acid media is eminently unsuited for excretion by animals whose urine is normally acid. Because of this insolubility the cystinuric man, although he may appear to be in perfect health, lives with the sword of Damocles suspended over his head. In Hutchinson's words, he has 'a peculiarity of health, giving proclivity to a definite form of disease'.

The special affliction of the cystinuric is the formation of urinary calculi, which in some instances attain to a large size, and in others are formed in very large numbers in the kidneys. In a few instances there have been found, in the bodies of young infants who have died in a marasmic state,* and some of whom were not known to be cystinuric during life, multiple deposits of crystalline cystin throughout the viscera.

Yet the cystinuric may go through life unaware of his peculiarity, and free from any calculous troubles. Thus several members of a family may all excrete cystine and show the deposits of hexagonal crystals in their urine, but it may be that only one of them will suffer from stones, and may form a number of stones in succession. It is obvious that there must be some external factor derived from the environment which thus discriminates between members of a family in all of whom the constitutional factor is present. Clearly the answer to be returned to the question what this influence is, has most important bearings upon the pathology of calculi in general.

Naunyn's work upon biliary calculi, and observations on cystinuric subjects, leads to the belief that it is to a local infection of the urinary tract, such as frequently occurs, that the inception of stone formation is to be ascribed. In the family of cystinurics the urine of the calculus-forming member alone may be infected with bacillus coli, but it must not be forgotten that such infection may be secondary to calculus formation. Some attempts, on Naunyn's lines, to find bacilli in a solution of the nucleus of a cystin calculus have hitherto failed, although the ready solubility of cystin in an alkali might be expected to facilitate such a search.

3482   o

* *young infants*   The disorder is probably infantile nephropathic cystinosis, an inborn error of lysosomal cystine efflux. It is a cause of the renal Fanconi syndrome.

Whether or no infection be the exciting cause, the anomaly under discussion offers an excellent example of a congenital defect, manifested in this instance by the formation of crystals in the urine and the development of serious morbid events under some external influence. Surely nothing can better fulfil the requirements of Ryle's [1] definition of a diathesis, 'a transmissible variation in the structure or function of tissues rendering them peculiarly liable to react in a certain way to certain extrinsic stimuli'.

There are very few[*] human cystinurics, possibly one in some thirty thousand living persons, and there are many sufferers from urinary calculi of various kinds. If the suggested factors are at work in the production of one species of calculus, like factors may be concerned in the production of stones of other kinds. The rare and exceptional example points out how such a result may be brought about, but it would, as yet, be rash to assume that other kinds of calculous disorders are attributable to like errors of metabolism.

The factor of insolubility of a metabolic product also plays an important part in connexion with the pathogeny of gout, a malady which found a place in every list of diathetic disorders, and might be described as the diathetic malady *par excellence*.

Around it was built up the whole conception of arthritism, the most viable of the diatheses of our forefathers, and that based upon the most imposing array of

[1] *Guy's Hosp. Gaz.*, 1926, xl. 546.

* *very few* The actual incidence in European populations is about twice Garrod's estimate.

facts. As the knowledge of gout goes back to the beginnings of medicine, so also does the recognition of its hereditary transmission. We all know of families some members of which develop gout at unusually early ages, and which include many victims of the malady. Thus, a man whose father and paternal grandfather had both suffered severely, had his first attack of orthodox gout in the great toe at the age of twenty. His two brothers and three sisters all suffered from true gout, and a son of one of his sisters had gout at the age of sixteen, whilst a schoolboy. This is, of course, a very extreme example. It would seem that if gout is inherited as a Mendelian characteristic, it is a dominant one. It is a matter of common experience that gouty attacks are much less often seen to-day than was the case fifty years ago, and this is as true of hospital practice as of that amongst people in more comfortable circumstances. This cannot be wholly explained by a change of fashion in nomenclature, in consequence of which many cases which would have formerly been called gouty, are assigned to other classes, and it would rather appear that changes of diet and modes of life render the exciting causes of the manifestations of gout less prevalent.

The study of the pathogeny of gout is beset with peculiar difficulties, and despite all the work which has been expended upon it since the detection of uric acid[*] in the blood of gouty people in the middle of the last century, no outstanding advance towards the solution of the problem has been made. A concensus of opinion

---

[*] *uric acid*   The first measurement of uric acid in the blood of patients with gout was made in 1848 by Sir Alfred Baring Garrod, father of A. E. Garrod.

nowadays favours the view that the underlying trouble is a derangement of purin metabolism. Even if it should be proved that the accumulation of uric acid in the blood of gouty subjects is due to defective excretion by the kidneys, it may nevertheless result from a defect of purin metabolism, for the deficient excretion may be due to a shortcoming of the product to be excreted, rather than of the excreting organs.

It is a well-known fact that the excretion of endogenous uric acid is independent of changes of diet, but varies rather widely in different individuals; and a systematic study of the purin metabolism, and of the blood content of uric acid in members of gouty families from infancy upwards, might go far towards the elucidation of the nature of the malady. At present we have no such data to go upon.

If gout be due to an inborn error of metabolism, such as is here suggested, it cannot be looked upon as due, like other such errors, to a rare mutation which occasionally occurs *de novo*, but rather as based upon an alternative and slightly divergent path of metabolism met with in a large part of the total population. It is interesting to note that there appears to be a special liability of the male sex, not to be explained by the influence of diet and environment.

It is a matter of observation that some individuals fail to develop gout,* in spite of diligent cultivation of those faulty habits which are supposed to conduce to attacks; in other words some are unable to acquire gout,

---

* *fail to develop gout*   In pointing out that some people escape gout no matter how diligently they cultivate the habits that seem to precipitate it in others, Garrod is emphasizing that we owe our strengths and immunities, no less than our infirmities, to chemical individuality.

however much they may try to do so, whilst others cannot escape it, however hard they try not to provoke it. The comparatively late age at which, with few exceptions, the onset of the disease occurs suggests that the underlying error is not, in itself, seriously detrimental to its subjects, but that it renders them unduly susceptible to external influences. Unless such influences come into play the gouty man may escape the manifestations of his malady, and it can hardly be doubted that many who inherit the susceptibility do actually escape.

There is no conclusive evidence that uric acid and the urates as such exert any toxic influence upon the tissues, and there is strong evidence that the pathological vice of sodium biurate, like that of cystin, is its scanty solubility, and its tendency to be deposited in crystalline form in the tissues, and especially in cartilage. It is permissible to suppose that the conditions which ensure the holding in solution of the urate are, in the gouty subject, taxed to the full, and that a variety of external influences may precipitate attacks.

In a given community the prevalent mode of life and the environment undoubtedly influence the frequency of gouty attacks to a remarkable extent, but that does not imply that they influence the number of potentially gouty individuals in the community.

The manifestations of gout are much more frequently seen in cities than in rural areas, and the prevalence of the disease in imperial Rome, and in other cities in which much luxury prevails is a notorious fact; but it is not a disease of the rich alone, and in all classes its frequency fluctuates from time to time. In the London hospitals it used to be common enough, but is now uncommon, in them, and in its severe forms, rare. In the hospitals in Edinburgh it was hardly ever seen at a time when it was commonly seen in those in London.

There can be no doubt that what enters by the mouth may contribute to the causation of gouty attacks, even though some of the diatetic advice habitually given to gouty subjects rests upon but slender foundations. The effect of chronic lead-poisoning admits of no doubt, and the power to provoke attacks of some foods, rich in purin bodies (such as thymus gland) which increases the uric acid in the blood, is apparently well established.

That injury can originate attacks of gout in the parts injured is beyond doubt. Even unusually hard use of a part may suffice, and so small an injury as is inflicted by syringing the ear of a patient on the verge of an attack has been known to provoke acute gout of the pinna. A blow upon a joint will suffice, and a first attack elsewhere than in the metatarso-phalangeal joint of the great toe, usually selects a joint which has been the seat of injury at some previous time. Lowered resistance may be due to other causes; and an attack of gout in a hemiplegic man tends to involve the joints of the paralysed half of the body.

The very liability of the great-toe joints, which was equally pronounced when sandals were the ordinary footwear, may reasonably be ascribed to the fact that these are the only joints which are damaged in walking, but defects of footwear doubtless contribute.

If the views here put forward are sound, gouty persons are subjects during the intervals between their attacks in which they may feel quite well, to 'a peculiarity of health' which gives proclivity to that particular form of disease; and just as a cystinuric may form no calculi, a gouty subject may never suffer from an actual attack of gout. It may be well to emphasize that the malady under discussion here has been true uratic gout, characterized by the deposition of crystalline sodium biurate in the tissues; a malady of which tophi in the ears may serve as a warning signs and serve as sure guides to diagnosis.

Much less is heard now than formerly of that congeries of discomforts and ailments which were formerly loosely classed as gouty, but which are now referred to other categories. The more exact indications afforded by the estimation of uric acid in a few drops of blood may reveal the gouty nature of troubles the true origin of which had not been suspected, and on the other hand corrects much loose classification. Nevertheless it must be remembered that increase of uric acid in the blood results from other causes besides gout.

The onset of the familiar osteo-arthritis of later life, with its erosion of cartilages, eburnation of bones, and formation of osteophytes, is often attributed to an injury. This is especially the case with the hip-joint disease of elderly people. Other manifestations of the malady, such as Heberden's nodes on the terminal phalanges of the fingers and the so common implication of the carpo-metacarpal joint of the thumb, are less obviously of traumatic origin, unless we reckon as trauma the continual wear and tear of a long life.

Another recognized causal factor of lesions of this type is a lowering of the resistance of the articular structures as the result of lesions of the nervous system, which is the most conspicuous factor in connexion with Charcot's disease of the joints in tabetic subjects. Infection also, and especially prolonged insidious infection, probably plays a part in a number of cases, but it must be admitted that in many cases of osteo-arthritis of the elderly no underlying cause can be recognized, whereas in some cases at any rate, the underlying factor is an inborn error of metabolism.

It was long supposed that the very rare error of protein metabolism, known as alcaptonuria, gave rise to no evil effects upon its subjects, beyond slight inconvenience due to the staining property of the urine. It is now recognized that this is not the case, but that the ill effects had been overlooked, because they are long delayed.

Alcaptonuria is characterized by blackening of the urine on exposure to air,* and the deep staining of fabrics moistened with the urine. These are the warning signals, and by their means it has been possible to trace back the anomaly to the first days of the life of its subjects. It is undoubtedly hereditary and inborn.

From the standpoint of heredity it behaves as a

* *blackening* A sign compatible with facilities for domestic sanitation prevalent in Garrod's time, likely to be missed with the modern flush toilet, visible again on the infant's cloth diaper deposited in a hamper, and again disappearing with the disposable diaper!

Mendelian recessive, appearing in several children of parents who are usually normal, and of whom a large proportion are consanguineous, usually first cousins. The proportion of consanguineous parents is far greater than in the population at large.

The essential error is apparently a failure to effect the complete catabolism of the tyrosin and phenyl-alanin contained in the proteins of the food and tissues, and the consequent presence of an intermediate product of the metabolism of these aromatic fractions of proteins. The product in question, homogentisic acid, or hydroquinone-acetic acid, shares with many other similar aromatic compounds the property of blackening on oxidation, and hence the characteristic property of alcapton urine.

In the course of years the homogentisic acid in the tissues brings about a selective blackening of certain tissues, notably of the articular and aural cartilages, and so is induced a condition first recognized in the cadaver by Virchow as one of extreme rarity, and called by him ochronosis. Albrecht was the first to suggest that alcaptonuria might be a cause of ochronosis, and Osler described clearly the clinical picture of the condition as seen in several elderly alcaptonurics under his observation. These observations have been abundantly confirmed, and the blue coloration of the interior of the ears, due to the black cartilage showing through the skin, the presence of brown triangular patches on the sclerotics, and occasionally pigmentation of the skin of the face, have been observed repeatedly in alcaptonurics over the age of thirty years.

The blue colour in the ears, and in some cases over the knuckle-joints, may be compared to the blueness of the sclerotics with brittleness of bones; but in one case the underlying tissues are stained, and in the other the overlying tissues are too transparent. The cartilages of a subject of ochronosis are raven black.

A closely similar ochronosis is produced in patients who have for many years applied carbolic dressings to ulcers, and, as far as is known, the alcaptonuric and the carboluric are the only varieties of ochronosis.

Ochronosis, in itself, may cause some disfigurement, only noticeable in extreme cases; but the alcaptonuric, as he grows older, tends to develop a form of osteo-arthritis, which is obviously intimately connected with the metabolic trouble. Hitherto no such association of osteo-arthritis with carbolic ochronosis has been observed, which is hardly remarkable seeing that in such ochronotics the cause has been at work for a much shorter time than in the lifelong alcaptonuric.

It might be suggested that the osteo-arthritis of later life is so common that the observed association with alcaptonuria may well be accidental, but such an interpretation is ruled out by two facts. Firstly, that, as in a family which Umber observed, in a sibship of several brothers and sisters, some alcaptonuric and others not, the articular lesions tend to occur in the alcaptonuric members only; and secondly, what is still more con-

clusive, the osteo-arthritis of alcaptonuria with ochronosis assumes a characteristic distribution and character
which has been observed in all the recorded cases. So
much is this the. case that its presence might be recognized by one who knows, from the peculiar stance
and gait of the sufferer.

The patient stands upon a wide base, and adopts a
stooping attitude, due, as Söderberg has pointed out, to
affection of the articulations of the spinal column. On
the other hand it has been shown that there may be
complete blackening of cartilages before there are any
anatomical changes in the joints; and the signs of
ochronosis become apparent to the clinical observer at
a considerably earlier period than those of implication
of the articular structures.

It would be wholly premature to suggest that the
presence of an unusual chemical compound in the
tissues and blood is the underlying factor in all cases of
osteo-arthritis, but it seems clear that in some instances
it is so, and that the lifelong presence of such a compound may produce its morbid effects only after the
lapse of many years.

Among the exciting causes of disease a not unimportant place must be assigned to light, and at the
present time when the beneficial action of light and
ultra-violet radiation are attracting so much attention,
it is well to be reminded that there are some to whom
bright light is a poison, and that there is a class of
maladies rightly named light diseases. One such is of

special interest in connexion with the subject of this chapter.

It is becoming increasingly evident that light and radiation beyond the wave-lengths of the visible spectrum exercise an important influence upon the vital processes of the animal organism, and as a conspicuous example may be quoted the action of light upon ergosterol, the production thereby of vitamin D, and the control so exerted upon the development of rickets. Again, it is known that human races differ markedly in their sensitivity to radiant energy, and that there have been evolved certain mechanisms for protection, such as pigmentation of the skin, and, what is less often seen, the growth of protective hair.

Furthermore, it has been shown that the introduction into the tissues of certain pigmentary compounds, mostly, if not all, fluorescent, of which eosin is an example, may render an individual acutely sensitive to light.

Amongst such substances the pigments of the porphyrin group, at least such of them as are fluorescent, hold prominent places; and of recent years much has been learnt of the nature and formation of those pigments.

In addition to haematoporphyrin, a pigment formed by the action of powerful reagents upon haemoglobin or haematin, we are now confronted with a whole group of porphyrins which differ more in their molecular structure than in the colour of their solutions and in their absorption spectra in acid and alkaline solutions respectively. They appear to be precursors, rather than

derivatives of haematin and haemoglobin, and to have
preceded the blood pigments in the evolutionary chain.
Moreover, they are to be obtained from vegetable as
well as animal sources, and even from yeast.

A pigment of this group, called by Hans Fischer
copro-porphyrin, because he first identified it in faeces,
is present in minute traces in the urine of normal human
beings; and it is tempting to imagine that similar traces
present in the tissues of the average man may play an
important part in connexion with the physiological
action of waves of short length.

Following the administration of certain drugs*over
long periods, of which drugs sulphonal has been the
chief offender, there occasionally develops a form of
acute poisoning, often fatal, of which the excretion of
porphyrins, in quantity sufficient to colour the urine a
deep red or brown, is a conspicuous sign. Curiously
enough the patients are almost always women. A
similar, but less fatal porphyrinuria is seen occasionally
as a symptom of disease, apart from the use of drugs.
Except in a case recorded by Haxthausen in which
luminal had been taken over a long period, and the red
urine was also of some standing, no skin affection due to
exposure to light has been observed in such cases, in
which the porphyrinuria is usually transient, or merely
an event in a fatal illness.

In some rare instances porphyrins are present in
abundance in the urine and faeces from birth onwards.
The dark red urine is the warning sign of this anomaly,

* *certain drugs* Garrod anticipates 'pharmacogenetics' (Motulsky 1957;
Vogel 1959); he called it 'idiosyncrasy' (see Garrod 1902, also *Inborn factors in
disease*, pp. 132, 155).

[141]

and it is fortunate that it is so rare; for the lot of its victims is indeed a deplorable one. It is probable that if they could live a troglodyte life, protected from any but subdued light, nothing serious would happen to them; it is when they are exposed to bright light that their troubles begin.

The recorded cases are not yet sufficiently numerous to justify dogmatic statements about its hereditary transmission, but so far as they go they point to such congenital porphyrinuria being a Mendelian recessive character. Several brothers and sisters have been affected born of parents apparently normal, and in several cases the parents of the sufferers have been first cousins. There is also the same predominance of males as with the other anomalies here discussed.

The subjects of congenital porphyrinuria develop, especially with the onset of summer, a form of skin eruption known as hydroa vacciniforme upon the exposed parts of the body, the face, the hands, and if they are uncovered, the knees. The eruption recurs, year after year, and leaves behind it cumulative scarring, and loss of substance in the parts attacked. Curiously enough, some parts of the face, and especially the chin, are seldom attacked.

Pigment is almost always deposited in the affected skin, as if to protect it from the light, and in a few cases there has been a profuse growth of hair, apparently for the same purpose. In some cases adult patients have exhibited most grave disfigurement, loss of substance of

the ears·and nose and even blindness from the implication of the cornea in the eruption. Nor is that all; the
deeper tissues also are affected, and there result deformities of the hands with stiffness of the fingers and
atrophy of the terminal phalanges. Another remarkable
effect is deep staining of the bones, and in some cases of
the milk teeth, and also those of the second dentition, by
porphyrin.

On the other hand it seems certain that porphyrinuria is not the only cause* of hydroa vacciniforme, any
more than alcaptonuria is the only cause of osteo-arthritis, nor that it is even its commonest cause. In cases
clinically similar there has been no excess of porphyrin
in the urine; but it is significant that when cases of
hydroa are collated both the sex incidence and type of
heredity in the whole series resemble closely those of the
porphyrinuric cases when taken alone. It may well be
that the cases without porphyrinuria have their origin in
some other metabolic error, or in several such, and that
the sensitivity of porphyrinurics to light is only a particular instance of a much wider phenomenon.

The light-sensitizing power of the porphyrins has
been proved by Hausmann and others by experiments
on mice and on protozoa, and by the daring experiment
of Mayer Betz upon himself, but hitherto it has proved
difficult to reproduce the exact conditions needed for
the development of the particular skin-eruption hydroa
vacciniforme.

Just as it is possible to produce a form of ochronosis

---

* *not the only cause* Garrod shows here, as elsewhere in the book, an open
mind, a willingness to embrace what we now call heterogeneity. In his time,
most physicians preferred to fit what they observed into some already well-
described pattern. He, in contrast, was always prepared to see something new.

by prolonged absorption of minute doses of carbolic acid, so a sensitivity to light, similar to that due to porphyrins, can be brought about by certain chemical substances taken by the mouth, such as eosin, or by certain articles of food such as buckwheat.

In his address of 1855, already referred to, Walshe not only suggested that diathetic diseases are apparently generated and sustained by an intrinsic blood-poison resulting from some perversion of the nutritive processes of the individual, but with equal prescience remarked that they resemble more or less closely the effects of certain inorganic poisons in small doses. Except that the poisons here discussed have been organic, not inorganic, Walshe's observation has a curiously modern ring. In the states which form the subject of this chapter there is present in the tissues an unusual chemical product, or a normal metabolic product in unusual amounts.

Its presence is apparently due to an arrest of metabolism, or to a deflexion of the metabolic path, probably due in either instance to the lack of an enzyme, of which the allotted task remains unperformed. Just as the deprivation of a vitamin, or the lack of a hormone, may bring about untoward results, so it would seem that the mere deficiency of an enzyme may be the underlying cause of morbid developments.

Albinism almost certainly results from a lack of the enzyme which produces melanin, and a still more striking example is afforded by that grave and remarkable malady haemophilia, a typical sex-limited recessive character, and, as such, difficult to eradicate from a stock. It can hardly be doubted that this is due to the absence of an enzyme concerned with the coagulation of the blood.

It might be objected that the conditions spoken of in this chapter are extremely rare, and that it is unsafe to draw any conclusions from them as to pathogeny in general. Yet if it be granted that every human being has his chemical individuality, as well as his individuality of form, we may well suppose that, seeing how conspicuous are the effects of the more pronounced departures from chemical type, the minor differences between any two of us may play important if less conspicuous parts as inborn factors in disease.

As was mentioned, Gaucher's disease may form a connecting link between tissue defects and inborn metabolic errors, and it is clear that a chemical defect may bring in its train highly selective damage to particular kinds of tissues.

There can be little doubt that, as time goes on, more and more inborn errors of metabolism will be brought to light; but it is to be hoped that a too ready application of that term will be avoided. There is danger lest it should be employed without any adequate reasons, and to quote Germain Sée once more, as merely 'un mot pour masquer notre ignorance'.

An important suggestion has been put forward by A. Hurst,[1] namely, that constitutional achlorhydria,

[1] *Brit. Med. Jour.*, 1927, i. 866.

which is met with even in young children, apart from obvious disease, and which tends to run in families, is an inborn error of secretion. This view is supported by the fact that such achlorhydria was detected, by Bennett and Ryle, in four out of a hundred healthy students, in the course of a systematic investigation of their gastric secretion. This opens up a new field of inquiry of great interest. If a like failure of secretion of endocrine glands could be established, this might explain much. How conspicuous the effects might be is shown in sporadic cretinism, where thyroid secretion fails owing to atrophy of the thyroid gland.

However this may be, the fact remains that in studying the chemistry of the individual as well as of the species, we get a clearer insight into the underlying, inborn factors in the pathogeny of some maladies. It may even be justifiable to claim that what our fathers called diathesis is only another name for chemical individuality.

VIII

THE INBORN FACTORS IN INFECTIVE DISEASES*

Der Leib der für die Infection immunen Thiere besitzt einen ihnen nicht zusagenden chemischen Bau, er ist chemisch anders beschaffen, als der jener Thiere deren Leib zur Wohnstätte der pathogenen Mikroorganismen geeignet ist.—H. HUPPERT, 1896.

IN the maladies hitherto considered the inborn factors play the more conspicuous parts, and in some of them, such as the neuromuscular abiotrophies, the

* *Infective diseases* In facing the issue of hereditary susceptibility to infections, Garrod was carrying the attack right to the citadel of the adversary; infections are the archetype of 'environmental' disease.

nature of the external factors is obscure. There are, on the other hand, many diseases in which the position is reversed, and the external factors are the most obvious and best defined. Without the tubercle bacillus there can be no tuberculosis, and without the plasmodium no malaria.

Nevertheless it must never be forgotten that it is not only in causing predisposition that internal factors are concerned; but also, that upon the patient's constitution depends the form* which the morbid syndrome assumes. As Sydenham[1] wrote, nearly three hundred years ago: 'a disease, however much its cause may be adverse to the human body, is nothing more than an effort of Nature, who strives with might and main to restore the health of the patient by the elimination of the morbific matter.'

The exogenous diseases,† as they may be called, are the most important of maladies, for they are responsible for the great bulk of human sickness, and for the largest part of the death-roll. In any medical ward in a hospital sufferers from infective diseases occupy most of the beds, and of such maladies tuberculosis, in its various forms, rheumatic fever and its sequels, and the troubles attributable to the pneumococcus and the streptococci are most abundantly represented. So it has come about that, in recent years, the importance of the parts played

[1] Medical Observations concerning the History and Cure of Acute Diseases (*Works of Thomas Sydenham*, translated by R. G. Latham, 1848, i. 29).

* *the form* · When the focus is upon external causes of disease, it may be forgotten how much the host influences the *form* a disease takes.

† *exogenous diseases* In one of the few reviews of The *inborn factors of diseases* (*British Medical Journal* 1932b) the writer remarks appropriately that improvement in public health had increased the relevance of constitutional diathesis in the pathogenesis of disease. At least someone got the message.

by the inborn factors has been, to a great degree, overlooked.

In our fight against the infective diseases*we are not confronted with blind forces, acting at random, but with the disciplined offensive of highly trained foes. Whilst on the one hand the weapons of attack have been improved by evolution, there has been a corresponding evolution of protective mechanisms of great ingenuity, and of no small efficiency, for the defence of the individual attacked. Against the production of the toxin must be set that of the antitoxin. We may suppose that in a large proportion, or even in the majority of instances, the attack fails, and the defensive forces win the day, even though the enemy may have effected a landing. As witness the large number of persons dying of other maladies in whose bodies are to be found extinct foci of tuberculosis. The chances of successful attack doubtless depend largely upon the nature and virulence of the attacking organism, as well as upon the immunity of the patient.

It follows that what we speak of as immunity is a positive quality, the possession of the power to produce antibodies, or the presence thereof in the organism. Predisposition to infective disease on the other hand is a negative characteristic, a lack of defensive substances or failure to produce them.

As yet we know but little†of the actual nature of compounds concerned in conferring immunity, nor how far biophysical as well as biochemical factors are con-

---

* *infective diseases* An infection is a consequence of the interaction of two chemical individualities—that of the micro-organism and that of the human host. Garrod's insight in this context has been amply supported and enlarged. There are perhaps 80 inborn errors of the immune-defence system and a molecular basis for both host susceptibility and microbial virulence is well established for many infections.

cerned in their working. Most of them are known to us only by single properties; just as for many years the element helium was known to us only by its line in the yellow of the solar spectrum, and adrenalin only by its effect upon blood-pressure.

It is not even certain whether the formation of an antibody is a chemical reaction which follows inevitably from the entrance into the body of a certain antigen; just as effervescence results whenever an acid is added to a solution of a carbonate; or whether the chemical reaction involved has been elaborated by an age-long process of evolution, to meet the special emergency when it arises.

The investigator engaged upon the synthesis of organic compounds can confidently expect that if he follows a certain line of procedure he will obtain a compound the properties of which he can foretell, although it may never previously have existed. So also, when a harmful aromatic compound enters the human body it is combined with sulphuric acid, and excreted as a harmless aromatic sulphate, and when an acid is administered to a carnivorous animal it is neutralized by ammonia, whereas in a vegetivorous animal, whose food is rich in fixed alkali, this mechanism is not required to protect the fixed alkalies of the tissues, and has not, apparently, been developed.

On the other hand, when Baumann administered brom-benzene to a dog the animal excreted a mercapturic acid, a derivative of cystin, and in this form got

---

† *know but little* (p. 124 Garrod's text)   This is illuminating of Garrod's always ranging mind. Where most are content to recount what is already known as if it were sufficient, Garrod invariably sees it as indicative of what is yet to be learned.

rid of the poison in question. The chemical reaction was ready to hand, but it is hard to believe that it had been evolved to meet the contingency; indeed it is unlikely that any dog had taken brom-benzene or other halogen-benzene previously. It is probable that some such reactions are prepared and others inevitable.

If this be true of immunity reactions also, it is possible that inborn immunity, when present, may be of the latter kind.

It is well known that animals of certain species are immune from certain infections to which members of other species are liable; it is also known that different races of men differ in their liabilities and immunities, and it is permissible to suppose that similar differences of lesser degree will be met with amongst individual human beings. Huppert[1] suggested, more than thirty years ago, that the differences between the species in this respect are due to their chemical build, which renders some better and some less favourable culture media for particular bacteria. In other words that resistance to this or that infection may be a fundamental property of the organism which exhibits it, but is as much a product of evolution* as its shape and size.

Seeing that attacks of many infectious diseases confer an immunity which may last for years, or even throughout life, it is, of necessity, no easy matter to distinguish between immunity which is inborn and that which has been acquired. The difficulty is aggravated by the fact

[1] *Die Erhaltung der Arteigenschaften*, 1896, p. 17.

* *product of evolution* Here Garrod is guessing, correctly, that the immune system has evolved to accommodate antigens never previously encountered by any species. This is a profound thought.

that we are constantly exposed to infections which fail to produce illness, but nevertheless call into play the protective mechanisms to counter them, with the result that a greater or less degree of immunity is acquired by individuals who are unaware that they have been exposed to the specific infection concerned. Furthermore, it is well established that maternal antibodies in the circulation of infants may confer an immunity during the early months of an infant's life. Consequently, when it is attempted to differentiate true inborn, or natural, immunity from such immunity as has been acquired after, or even before, birth the inquirer is in like position to one who listens to a wireless programme which is seriously obscured by heterodyne transmissions.

There is strong evidence that a community may acquire, in the course of time, a relative immunity from an infection to which it has been long and continuously exposed; whereas another community,* not so protected by secular exposure, may, when the disease in question is introduced into it, suffer in wholesale numbers and from attacks of extreme severity and fatality. This may be due to acquired immunity produced by continual minor infections, or, as some think, and as Archdall Reid[1] so strongly urged, to raising of the level of protection by the weeding out†of the more susceptible members by natural selection.

The clinical evidence of the existence of inborn im-

[1] *The Laws of Heredity,* 1910.

* *another community* It is generally agreed now that such populations do not differ genetically from others. Rather it is that the diseases are milder in the children of populations where they are endemic and so do not show the mortality observed in a previously unexposed population.

† *weeding out* Survivors of epidemics of infantile diarrhoea in two New England villages were shown, on average, to outlive their controls who had not been exposed to the epidemics (Meindl 1982).

munities from and liabilities to infective maladies is very strong, and is convincing to the family medical attendant who watches his patients and their families over long periods of years. There are families in which various members develop, at different times, and in different environments, in circumstances which exclude infection of member by member, such a disease as typhoid fever. In some families scarlet fever is unknown, despite frequent exposures of some of its members to infection. The experience of many of us suggests that when, after many years of absence, influenza returned in pandemic form some forty years ago, different individuals showed very different degrees of susceptibility to the infection.

In weighing such clinical evidence it is necessary to bear in mind that what appears to be a familial suscepti-bility to an infective malady may, in reality, be the out-come of direct infection of member by member. This source of error was particularly active in connexion with tuberculosis, in days when the bacterial origin and infective character of that disease were as yet unsus-pected. In houses often deliberately ill-ventilated, one after another of the younger members of a family 'went into a decline' as the saying was; and in some instances years elapsed between the deaths of the infecting and infected members.

Only when cases are carefully watched, and the sources of error are excluded as far as possible, can the strength of the clinical evidence be estimated. Statis-tical inquiries* yield very valuable checks. As was men-

---

* *Statistical inquiries* Textbooks of medicine of Garrod's time refer to familial propensities for, as well as possible resistance to, particular infections. But few of Garrod's colleagues urged testing of such distinctions by 'statistical inquiries'.

tioned in an earlier section, the statistical investigations of the incidence of tuberculosis by Karl Pearson, Stocks, and Govaerts show a somewhat higher incidence of that disease in individuals in whose family it has occurred in previous generations, than in those whose family history presents a clean bill of health in that respect.

Obviously a definite test of susceptibility to infection offers the best chance of gaining reliable information regarding the existence or otherwise of inborn natural immunity to infective maladies, and in this connexion Schick's test of liability to diphtheria holds out the greatest promise of usefulness. If it can be shown that immunity from diphtheria conforms to some definite scheme of heredity, such evidence will be of special importance, for the risk of confusion with acquired immunity will be excluded. However, in the opinion of some who are well qualified to judge, the response to the question which the Schick test supplies is not unequivocal.

The test in question indicates the presence in the blood or tissues of the individual to whom the test is applied of diphtheria antitoxin, or at least his power of producing the antitoxin with ease.

H. and L. Hirszfeld[1] have carried out an elaborate investigation upon a large number of families and of individuals, both with the Schick test and with the Dick test of susceptibility to scarlet fever. These in-

[1] *Klin. Wchnschr.*, 1924, iii. 2084; *Ztschr. f. Immunitätsforsch.*, 1927–8, liv. 81; *Lancet*, 1919, ii. 675.

vestigators found a connexion* between Schick liability
and the blood groups of the individuals tested; and
from this conclude that diphtheria immunity, which is
thus correlated with factors which are definitely constitutional, cannot depend upon external influences alone,
but must have a constitutional basis. They found that
if one parent be Schick positive and the other negative,
the children with the same blood group as the positive
parent are themselves positive, whereas those which share
the blood group of the negative parent are themselves
negative for the most part, although some are not so.

As regards the Schick test the Hirszfelds find that
when both parents give positive reactions, in other
words are liable to acquire diphtheria because they are
poor producers of antitoxin, almost all their offspring
are positive also, as might be expected with a Mendelian
recessive factor. On the other hand if both parents are
negative, i.e. have the power of forming antitoxin well
developed, some one-third of the offspring are positive
and the remaining two-thirds negative, in other words
are either apparent or actual dominants. Again, when
one parent is positive and the other negative about half
the children are positive and half negative.

To avoid confusion it must be borne in mind that
what is positive in Schick terminology is, in Mendelian
terms, a negative factor, namely lack of power to form
antitoxin, whereas a Schick negative reaction implies
a positive characteristic, namely the possession of such a
power.

* *connexion*   The Hirszfelds' 'connexion' between response to the Schick
test and the ABO blood group system must be among the first (perhaps the
first) examples of associations of a sort that are turning up with increasing
frequency now. The association of HLA alleles with autoimmune diseases is
now well known.

Here also are traces of that enigmatical sex-linkage, such as is seen in the metabolic errors, but in this instance the advantage lies with the males, who are less liable than females.

Clinical evidence points to a greater liability to diphtheria of females, and observations with the Schick test tend to confirm that impression. There is similar support for the belief, based upon clinical observation, that some races of mankind are more liable than others to acquire diphtheria.

S. F. Dudley,[1] in a critical review of the whole subject in which the findings with the Schick test, and the inferences based upon them, are subjected to a searching criticism, writes as follows: 'The evidence on the whole seems to favour the hypothesis that the potentiality of responding to antigenic stimuli from the diphtheria bacilli in the environment is greater in the average male than the average female. If this be so, susceptibility to diphtheria is to some extent a real, hereditary, sex-linked character.'

Again: 'A general survey of the evidence does undoubtedly suggest that a small percentage of the population are born with genetic defects in their potentiality to form diphtheria antitoxin, but that this hereditary factor has an insignificant bearing on the degree of immunity possessed by a community as a whole, compared with the concentration, distribution, and persistence of diphtheria bacilli in the environment.'

[1] *Quart. Jour. Med.*, 1928–9, xxii. 321.

It may be pointed out that the frankly infectious maladies had no place in the lists of diathetic diseases compiled in the last century, and when the difficulty of discriminating the inborn factors amidst so many obscuring influences is taken into account their omission need cause no surprise. The lists did include some maladies due to bacterial infection, such as tuberculosis and leprosy, but in those days it was not suspected that either of those maladies was contagious.

As regards the influence of the individuality of the patient upon the clinical picture of the infective diseases there is not much that can be said. The effect of the age of the patient upon the clinical picture of rheumatic fever has been referred to, but as a rule it is difficult to say whether a peculiarity in response to an invasion is due to a peculiarity in the invading organism, or in the patient. There can be little doubt that many of the signs of the exanthemata are allergic in their nature, and in their allergic responses individuals differ widely; how widely is shown in the conditions known as idiosyncrasies, which will form the subject of the chapter which follows.

IX

IDIOSYNCRASIES

Idiosyncrasy is individuality run mad.—JONATHAN HUTCHINSON.

NO discussion of the inborn factors in disease would be at all complete which left out of account the conditions commonly spoken of as idiosyncrasies.*

* *idiosyncrasies* Garrod, as usual, avoids self-citation. Anyone who has not yet read his earlier paper (Garrod 1902) should do so. It is nominally about alcaptonuria; it is actually about 'idiosyncrasis', diathesis, and above all human chemical individuality.

Strictly speaking the term idiosyncrasy should be used to cover the whole ground of our individual differences, as co-extensive with our personalities. Jonathan Hutchinson, in his *Pedigree of Disease*, includes under the name even such structural anomalies as coloboma of the iris and cleft palate, and H. D. Rolleston,[1]*in a recent monograph on idiosyncrasies, includes a psychological group, in which an idea or emotion, such as does not upset the average†man or woman, brings about most unexpected reactions.

The peculiarities here to be considered cover a much more limited field, for in medical parlance the name idiosyncrasy is commonly applied to exceptional responses, on the part of exceptional individuals, to stimuli which are insufficient to produce any conspicuous effects in the great majority of members of the human race. Such stimuli are often applied in the forms of articles of diet or particular drugs, the pollen of particular plants, or the exhalations of particular animals.

Rolleston defines an idiosyncrasy as 'an abnormal reaction in an otherwise normal person, which may be either, on the one hand, greatly exaggerated, or, on the other hand, greatly diminished; more briefly it may be described as an unusual physiological personal equation'. The inclusion in this definition of what may be called negative idiosyncrasies is of special interest. It can hardly be doubted that there are variations to both sides of the average line, and that there are persons who

[1] *Idiosyncrasies*, 1927.

* *Rolleston* The co-author of a contemporary textbook of medicine (Allbutt and Rolleston 1910), and the author of a book on idiosyncrasy (Rolleston 1927).

† *the average* There is no single normal homeostatic value. Populations have dispersion of values about the central tendency—or homing value in a regulated system (Murphy and Pyeritz 1986). Outlier values may indicate predisposition, with an idiosyncratic response, to a perturbing stimulus.

respond less vigorously to the stimuli mentioned than do the bulk of human beings. However, we should expect that such negative idiosyncrasies would be more difficult to study than are the converse positive peculiarities.

The idiosyncrasies are of special importance from the point of view set out in this essay, for nowhere are our individualities more clearly manifested than in such wide departures from type.

Whereas we might hesitate to label an attack of giant urticaria, following the eating of honey, and recurring whenever honey be eaten, as a disease in the ordinary sense of that term, it is not possible to draw any sharp dividing line between such attacks and morbid pictures to which no one would hesitate to apply the name. Some varieties of asthma fall into the one, and some into the other category.

A large number, perhaps the largest number of idiosyncrasies, are manifestations of hypersensitiveness, and their symptoms are such as characterize allergic or anaphylactic states, which result from the introduction of foreign proteins into the organism.

Immunological investigations have shown that the intrusive substance, the so-called antigen, encounters, chiefly in the tissue cells, a substance which is antagonistic to it, an antibody, and to the effects of their encounter the observed phenomena are ascribed.

These symptoms differ in conspicuous ways in animals of different genera; the suffocative syndrome presented by the anaphylactic guinea-pig bears little outward resemblance to that manifested by an anaphylactic dog.

Anaphylaxis, properly so-called, is an artificial or adventitious state, which results from the injection of a protein into an animal which has previously been sensitized by the administration of a dose of the same protein. Nevertheless, certain of the symptoms which enter into the composition of the anaphylactic syndrome, such as rashes, usually urticarial, gastric disturbances, and respiratory embarrassment, are met with not only in anaphylactic states, but also in connexion with many of the human idiosyncrasies as regards drugs, foodstuffs, pollens, and animal emanations.

That some individuals are far more liable than average people to respond injuriously to such provocations is an undoubted fact, and it is reasonable to ascribe their sensitivity to the presence in their tissues of an antibody, ready to combine with the antigen when it comes their way. Indeed, Prausnitz and Kuster[1] detected such substances, which they called 'atopic reagins', in the blood of hypersensitive individuals, and by injecting blood from such an atopic individual into the skin of a normal man they rendered the injected area of the skin of the recipient, and that area alone, sensitive to the foodstuffs or pollens which gave rise to allergic reactions in the donors of the blood.

There is strong evidence that in the subjects of the

[1] *Zentralbl. f. Bakt., Abth. 1 (Originale)*, 1921, lxxxvi. 160.

allergic idiosyncrasies the hypersensitivities which they exhibit are inborn peculiarities in most, if not in all cases; nevertheless, as in not a few hereditary morbid conditions, their manifestations may be postponed, and may not be in evidence during the early years of life or even longer. Thus, an article of diet which was previously taken with impunity, may be found, in later life, to elicit an allergic response. Conversely it is undoubtedly the case that an idiosyncrasy to a particular antigen may disappear as an individual grows older, probably as the result of a process of desensitization.

There is a large amount of evidence of the hereditary transmission of hypersensitivities; but it would appear that members of different generations of a family, and even members of the same sibship of brothers and sisters, although hypersensitive, in the sense under discussion, do not always react exceptionally to the same antigens.

Cooke and van der Veer,[1] in America, found that hypersensitivity could be traced in the antecedents of 48·5 per cent. of a group of 504 individuals who themselves exhibited some form of hypersensitivity, but in the antecedents of only 14·5 per cent. of normal individuals. The same investigators found that the allergic symptoms tended to make their first appearance between the ages of 20 and 26 years in persons having only one hypersensitive parent, whereas in children both of whose parents were hypersensitive, the symptoms appeared at 5 years or earlier.

[1] *Jour. Immunol.*, 1916, i. 201.

The hereditary transmission of hay-fever and of asthma is well recognized; angioneurotic oedema has been traced through five generations of a family in which the condition proved fatal in a number of cases, and even so highly specialized an idiosyncrasy as intolerance of egg-albumin has been recorded as occurring in three generations of a family.

The simplest of all forms of allergic idiosyncrasy is that known as 'factitious urticaria' or 'dermatography'. Here the exciting cause is no introduction of a foreign protein or other substance, but a mere mechanical pressure often of a very slight kind. Anything written or drawn upon the skin of a subject of this anomaly, even by gentle pressure with a pencil or other blunt point, stands out, after a short time, in the form of raised wheals. The phenomenon is an exaggeration of normal happenings, but provoked by a pressure which would cause but insignificant manifestations in an average individual.

The series of phenomena observed in subjects of factititous urticaria, and in less pronounced degree in average individuals, has formed the subject of a masterly investigation by Thomas Lewis[1] and his fellow workers. The initial flush, due to dilatation of capillaries, the more lasting flare around the seat of pressure, which is due to relaxation of the adjacent arterioles, and the eventual wheal, are also members of the anaphylactic syndrome, and are signs met with in a number of other

[1] *The Blood Vessels of the Human Skin, and their Responses*, 1927.

3482 S

kinds of idiosyncrasy, elicited by other causes than mere pressure.

Lewis, in the course of his work, has traced the production of the flush, flare, and wheal to the liberation by the injured cells of a substance which he calls the 'H substance'. This initial was chosen because of the similarity of the physiological action of the H substance to that of histamine, a base derived from histadine by removal of a CO_2 group, and which was originally found in the tissues by Dale and Barger. H. H. Dale[1] has since advanced strong reasons for taking a bolder view, and for the identification of the H substance with histamine, which base is known to be present normally in the tissues.

The expression 'liberation of histamine' is a somewhat guarded one, but it is more probable that, under the influence of agents which damage the tissue cells, the preformed histamine which they normally contain escapes into the circulation, than that histamine is formed in excess, as a result of the damage, and is thrown out for any protective purpose.

Seeing that the same triple response, the flush, the flare, and the wheal, figures amongst the anaphylactic reactions in healthy skins, Lewis came to the conclusion that the union of antigen and antibody in the cells in which it occurs liberates the preformed H substance, just as a mechanical injury does; and Dale regards this

[1] 'Croonian Lectures on some Chemical Factors in the Control of the Circulation', *Lancet*, 1929, i. 1285.

explanation as accounting for all the known facts. He
points out that by any of the earlier conceptions of the
process at work, it was difficult to explain why, in each
species of animal, only those cells which are normally
sensitive to histamine appear to be sensitive also to the
foreign antigen, and respond to its injection.

If Lewis's explanation be adopted this need not be
assumed. It is only necessary to suppose that from
whichever cells histamine may be set free, by the union
of antigen with antibody within them, those cells which
are normally sensitive to histamine take part in the
production of the obvious reaction which results.

On this theory we have not to deal with an undue
sensitivity of certain cells to histamine, but with excessive liberation of that substance, either into the parts
adjacent to the seat of its liberation, or when, as in the
dog, the setting free of histamine results from anaphylactic damage to a large viscus, such as the liver, the
discharge is into the general blood-stream. So it comes
about that the liberated histamine produces its characteristic response in cells which are normally sensitive to
that base, but which are not themselves affected by
the antigen. In this way may be explained the striking
differences in the anaphylactic syndrome, as seen in
animals of different species, such as the dog and the
guinea-pig respectively.

As Dale points out further: 'We may picture the
anaphylactic shock, therefore, as the result of cellular
injury due to the intra-cellular reaction of the antigen

with an aggregating antibody. Whether this is general, or localized in a particular organ, histamine will be released, and its effects will be prominent in the resulting reaction; imposing a general resemblance to the syndrome produced by histamine itself on the symptoms seen in each species.' In this way it is possible to explain the likenesses and the differences of the anaphylactic attacks in animals of different species.

So also it is possible to 'explain the effects of the various "allergens" or "haptenes" on a subject of a natural or acquired idiosyncrasy. Whatever view be taken as to the similarities or differences between such conditions and artificial anaphylaxis, all certainly involve a condition of the cells such that a normally harmless substance is specifically injurious to them; in all cases the reaction to such a specific injury involves symptoms like those produced by histamine, and for the reason that in all cases histamine is released by the injury'.

It follows that the histamine syndrome cannot be regarded as peculiar to anaphylaxis, seeing that it may be produced by the liberation of histamine owing to various causes; in a very sensitive individual by so slight a mechanical insult as pressure of a pencil point upon the skin. Nor is it surprising that the necessary cellular injury may be brought about by other than protein compounds, such as quinine and antipyrin.

It is obvious that although histamine produces some of the most conspicuous of the allergic symptoms, it is

[164]

no more the cause of anaphylaxis and allergy than gun-powder is the cause of war. An explanation has still to be sought for the extraordinary hypersensitiveness of the cells of certain individuals to injuries of certain kinds, and the readiness of those cells to set free histamine under provocation which fails to produce such results in the cells of the average man.

It is, at least, highly probable that the explanation of allergy is to be found in the chemical individuality of the subject, and of those of his cells which are damaged by antigen, seeing how discriminative is the action of the causative agents at work. If there were merely a greatly exaggerated sensitiveness to histamine of the cells which are normally sensitive to it but in a far lesser degree, we should expect that disturbance would be induced by any of the recognized causes of the histamine syndrome, from slight mechanical pressure upwards; but this is far from being the case. Therefore it must be assumed that the cells of a subject of facti-tious urticaria are not unduly sensitive to histamine, but that they liberate that substance with undue readiness, whereas in the great majority of human beings the histamine syndrome produced by pressure upon the skin is far less pronounced, and requires greater pres-sure for its induction.

As a rule, of the known causes of allergy only one is effective in any particular case.

It will be remembered that Cooke and van der Veer found that in families containing hypersensitive members, the exciting cause of the manifestations may not be the same in all the members, but in some cases sensitiveness to a particular antigen, such as egg albumin, is manifested by members of successive generations of a family. It would seem that the essential factor is the chemical or physico-chemical interplay of antigen and antibody in the cells of the subject, as the result of which histamine is liberated from the damaged cells. What is inherited is an undue liability to such cellular protests against some particular antigen or antigens, but not always the same ones.

Examples of such selective idiosyncrasies are quoted by all authors who have written upon the subject. The present writer, who has not, to his knowledge, any excessive sensitivity to any other flower or plant, and who does not suffer from hay-fever, is unable to stay in a room with the flowers of the orange-coloured buddleia without experiencing general discomfort and breathlessness, but without any stridor. The purple buddleia, on the other hand, has no such effect.

A member of a former generation of his family could not, when young, eat any fish of the family of the pleuronectidae, sole, plaice, turbot, halibut, and the like, without experiencing severe gastric symptoms; but from middle life to extreme old age, she could eat such fishes without ill effect.

All men are subject to some allergic effects, upon adequate provocation, and it would be difficult to suppose that whereas some are much more sensitive than the average man, there are not others who are decidedly less sensitive. It is naturally more difficult to bring forward examples of such negative idiosyncrasies; but perhaps the best known is the scanty response of some individuals to bites of such insects as fleas and to the stings of nettles.

From a mere idiosyncrasy towards a particular antigen there are all stages to what are known as the allergic diseases; of which asthma is the most important, although angio-neurotic oedema is more fatal. Such diseases have been discussed widely in recent years, on the Continent by Storm van Leeuwen,[1] in this country by Hurst,[2] and in America by Coca,[3] Cooper, and others.

Idiosyncrasies to drugs are sometimes of the allergic kind, as when a drug such as quinine or antipyrine gives rise, whenever taken, to an urticarial rash, with or without attendant vomiting. In some cases a drug produces an effect quite unlike its usual action, as when opium causes excitement; but more usually the normal action of the drug is induced by unusually small doses, or on the other hand an abnormal degree of tolerance may be manifested.

Every drug which has a definite physiological action acts as a poison when taken in excessive doses, but in different individuals and in animals of different species

[1] *Allergic Diseases*, 1925.
[2] A. F. Hurst, *The Constitutional Factor in Disease*, 1927.
[3] Coca, *Essentials of Immunology*, 1925.

the dose per kilogram needed for the production of such effects differs omewhat*widely. The same is true of children and adult men and women respectively, as witness the well-known tolerance by children of belladonna, and their relative intolerance of opium.

Much experimental work has been carried out, by Clark[1] and others, upon the tolerance of drugs by animals, and a mass of evidence regarding this matter was brought together, in a critical review, by J. A. Gunn[2] in 1923. Some of the protective methods directed to saving the tissues from the ill effects of chemical poisons were spoken of in an earlier section, but it should be mentioned further that there is reason to believe that the destruction of drugs within the body is brought about in not a few cases by enzyme action; it would appear that in the cases of atropine, morphia, and strychnine amongst other alkaloids, the liver is the organ chiefly instrumental in their destruction. It may well be that, as Gunn suggests, the ferments concerned are usually occupied in dealing with ordinary products of metabolism, rather than that they lie in wait in the tissues in the hope that some day their appropriate alkaloid may come along.

It will have been seen that all that we know of the nature of idiosyncrasies, either allergic or other, suggests that the factors which bring about their manifestations are intimately connected with the chemical life of

[1] *Quart. Jour. Exper. Physiol.*, 1912, v. 385.
[2] *Physiol. Rev.*, 1915, iii. 41.

* *differs omewhat* Printer's error.

their subjects, and the chemical structure of their tissues. Their tendency to family occurrence, and their intimate relationship to such hereditary maladies as angioneurotic oedema and asthma, suggest strongly that idiosyncrasies are inborn peculiarities, even in cases in which they do not manifest themselves in the early years of life.

Epilogue

Mehr und mehr wirt die Krankheitslehre zur Konstitutionspathologie: zwar wirkt die Umwelt auf den Körper ein; aber Art und Grad der Wirkung hängt von der angeborenen Anlage ab.—WILHELM HIS. 1928.

THE subjects which have been touched upon in the course of this essay, as illustrating the importance and the nature of the inborn factors in disease, cover so wide a field, and throw light upon the subject from such different angles, that it will be well to take stock, in a brief concluding review, of the general conclusions arrived at or suggested, of the way in which the several pieces of the puzzle can be fitted together.

It was pointed out, in the historical introduction, how, starting from the recognition of morbid predispositions, there were built up theories of diatheses which assumed various forms, but which were all impaired by the lack of knowledge, in the days in which they were propounded, of fundamental problems upon which modern science has thrown fresh light. Hence it became obvious that in order to arrive at any sound conclusions on the liabilities of individuals to, and their immunity from certain maladies, it was necessary to approach the subject *de novo* in the light of that more recent knowledge, whilst recognizing fully that in fifty years*a still more ample knowledge will doubtless displace many of our own conclusions in turn.

The further nosology is pursued, the more clearly does it emerge that in every case of every malady there

* * *fifty years* The 50 years, far from displacing the conclusion (following paragraph), confirm it.

[170]

are two sets of factors at work in the formation of the morbid picture, namely internal or constitutional factors, inherent in the sufferer and usually inherited from his forebears, and external ones which fire the train. In some instances, and especially in infective diseases, the external factors dominate the picture, in so far as the causation of the trouble is concerned, but the symptoms observed represent the response of the patient to the assault of the invaders. In some other maladies, such as the hereditary abiotrophies of the neuromuscular system, the external factors are so little in evidence that they are apt to be overlooked. Between these two extremes various intermediate stages are met with.

The constitution of a man is the sum of *all* his qualities, his bodily form, the structure of his tissues, his coloration, height, weight, blood-pressure, and body temperature; as well as his mental and moral qualities, functional processes, and tricks of gesture and action.*

In all or some of these respects each man differs from all his fellows, for even uniovular twins are not exactly alike.

The differences between the various species of animals in their chemical build and chemical processes are well known, and it follows, and can indeed be demonstrated, that the individual members of a species are likewise possessors of chemical individuality; that each is built up of slightly different materials from his fellows, and leads his own chemical life. Seeing that all the factors in the constitution of the future man are represented in

* *constitution*   This idea of constitution was in common usage in Garrod's time. It was recognized by Hutchinson, Rolleston, Pearl, and others that people differ as a result of endowment and development. For example, there is a chapter on the subject (written by Hutchinson) in Allbutt and Rolleston's (1910) textbook of medicine. Pearl published a book called *Constitution and health* in 1933 and Hurst, *The constitutional factor in disease* in 1927. But none of these authors gave 'constitution' the chemical basis of which Garrod makes such a point, and which accounts for our current interest in him as opposed to them.

the chromosomes of the germinal cells from which he shall spring, it can hardly be supposed that such diverse potentialities as are foreshadowed in structures so minute, and so little different from each other as are the germinal cells of creatures of different species, can have other than a molecular representation.

If this be so, it can hardly be doubted that variations in the chemistry of the chromosomes of the germinal cells are the starting-points of mutations great and small. Upon these mutations natural selection is continually at work, ensuring the persistence of those which make for the welfare of the organism and the species, and weeding out those which are detrimental. It is even difficult to escape the conclusion that upon the chemical structure of the chromosomes depend even the structure and forms of the creatures which spring from them, and the anatomical deviations from type which some of them display. How profound an influence chemical products can exert upon form is shown in the workings of some of the hormones.

A particular mutation may recur, apart from inheritance, just as the same chemical reaction will be repeated whenever the same reagents come together under suitable conditions. We are not obliged to suppose that all those who exhibit a mutation, even a very rare one, are, to whatever the race they may belong, members of a single family.

On the other hand, it is because an individual is able to hand on to his descendants some favourable mutation which he has developed that improvement of the race is possible.

Many of the difficulties which surround the phenomena of heredity have been removed in recent years, and Mendel's theory serves to explain the skipping of one or more generations, the occurrence of an anomaly in several children of parents who are themselves apparently normal, and the remarkable sex-linked inheritance of haemophilia.

In the course of ages the human organism has become remarkably well adapted to the conditions in which it lives, and it is able to adapt itself to somewhat wide changes of environment; as witness man's power to live in the polar regions or in the tropics, on the mountain side or below the sea-level. Nevertheless, that condition of adjustment which we speak of as health is maintained only by a continuous struggle; it is a dynamic, not a static state, and there is truth in the popular phrase, for a man *keeps* rather than *remains* healthy.*

Man has to struggle against his own individual shortcomings upon the one hand, and against physical agents, chemical poisons, and the attacks of pathogenic organisms on the other hand.

What we describe as diseases are groups of symptoms, forming clinical and pathological pictures which portray that struggle. Many such pictures represent the reaction of the organism to the attacks of morbific agents; its attempts, which happily are often successful, to beat off or destroy the invaders.

* *a man keeps* . . .   We seem only recently to have learned this fact. Garrod would have been amused to see the joggers, the health spas, and the industries that cater to the 'continuous struggle' to keep healthy.

To every attack of invaders of the same species human beings tend to return the same reply, but slightly modified by their own idiosyncrasies; and such replies to specific infections are the characteristic pictures spoken of as measles, scarlet fever, variola, and the like. Some pathogenic organisms give rise to pictures which differ according to the parts attacked; such as the various kinds of illnesses due to the pneumococcus and tubercle bacillus respectively. Indeed the functions of organs or structures which become the seats of local lesions determine the shapes of many morbid pictures. This is particularly the case with lesions of nerve centres such as that which lies behind tabes dorsalis; and with those which upset the regulative balance of the endo-crine system, by inducing over-activity of a particular gland, as in Graves's disease, or suppression of its functions, as in myxoedema.

Yet other pictures portray the struggle of the organism to carry on its functions, although essential supplies from without are being witheld. The lacking supplies may be of oxygen, foodstuffs, water, or of the vitamins which, although needed in such small quanti-ties, play most essential parts in animal nutrition.

Obviously, pictures of such diverse kinds cannot be fitted into any truly systematic classification[*]; but many of them are met with so often, and under such constant guises, that they demand places in some scheme of classification; and indeed some such is essential for the study and teaching of clinical medicine.

[*] *systematic classification*   Garrod returns to the unsatisfactory systems of disease classification, and to the need for one 'for the study and teaching of clinical medicine'. We are no nearer such a classification today. A comparison of *Modern medicine* by Osler and McCrae (1925) with the current edition of Harrison's *Principles of Internal Medicine* (Petersdorf et al. 1983) shows that the latter relies upon the same classification by aetiology and organ system as the former.

Unquestionably disease has played, and is playing, a very important role in the process of evolution, and is a potent agent for the weeding out of those least able to survive. But as man has developed, the process of survival of the fittest, in Nature's sense, has received a check, as far as the human race is concerned. The ideals of mutual help, the care devoted to the maimed and mentally deficient, and indeed the entire arts of medicine and surgery, are marshalled in direct opposition to the struggle for existence, as it is seen in the lower animals. Clearly, it is to his brain rather than to his muscles that man owes his survival and his high place in Nature.

When we speak of a normal man we mean one who does not depart, in any conspicuous respect, from the average of the race. That average cannot be represented by a sharp line, but by a series of dots, some to one and some to the other side of an imaginary line. Some of us deviate from the normal to our benefit, and some of us to our detriment.

The various races of mankind, and groups of people who may, or may not, be descendants of common ancestors, show constitutional resemblances, including likenesses in face and form, as well as in mental qualities and dispositions. With these resemblances are often linked* degrees of liability to suffer from particular diseases. Hence the study of bodily form by anthropometric methods can give intimations of the maladies from which individuals are likely to suffer; but the peculiarities of outward form are in no sense the causes of disease,

* *linked*   Garrod appears to be referring here to a fad, current in his time but which soon lost acceptance: that of associating disease with bodily form and other outward characteristics. Draper was its principal exponent in America.

but are the labels indicative of particular morbid liabilities.

On the other hand, amongst the unnumbered differences of form which serve to distinguish each man from his fellows, there are some which may handicap him on his way through life, may lame him or disfigure him, and others which directly predispose him to disease. An abnormal mesentery may lead to strangulation of the intestine, an abnormal diverticulum may become the seat of inflammation or ulceration, a malformed cardiac valve may suffer too readily from infection. Yet such accidents are too uncommon to play any conspicuous parts in the aetiology of disease, nor is any important general inference to be drawn from them.

In some human families numbers of members exhibit anomalies of particular tissues, or tissues of certain groups, which are strongly suggestive of defects in the materials of which the affected tissues are constructed, or of the manner in which the materials are put together; as if Nature had descended to jerry-building. A conspicuous example is afforded by the highly hereditary kind of brittleness of bones, in which the defect of the connective tissues is made evident by undue translucency of the sclerotics which appear blue in colour because the black choroid shows through them. It is shown also in the fragility of the bones which are broken by slight injuries. Upon this congenital defect is engrafted, as time goes on, a progressive disease, otosclerosis.

[176]

In all probability minor defects of tissues are very common, and not only defects but also improvements upon the average standard. Various examples were alluded to in section vi of this essay. They are of widely different kinds, but in all some particular kind of tissue is implicated, and even when the trouble is not obvious at birth, that tissue appears to be unable to stand even the ordinary wear and tear of life. Of special interest are the maladies, hereditary, and sooner or later fatal, of the neuromuscular system, to which Gowers gave the name of abiotrophies. In them we see what Galton described as 'the steady and pitiless march of the hidden weaknesses in our constitutions through illness to death'.

Their subjects may appear to be in perfect health during their early years, and only show signs of their disease in later childhood, or even later. But their hereditary and family occurrence, which is specially well marked in that sex-linked recessive condition pseudo-hypertrophic muscular dystrophy, point clearly to an inborn defect. Although it is generally assumed that the tissues themselves are at fault in the abiotrophies, and that their power of resistance to the unavoidable minor accidents of life is so seriously impaired that, as Rosenbach put it, the ordinary use of the parts amounts to an injury, the possibility is not wholly excluded that the tissues involved may be damaged, or rendered sensitive to damage, by the presence in them of some metabolic product which progressively impairs their in-

tegrity. As yet there is little evidence in support of
either hypothesis. The changes observed in the
apparently unaffected muscles of dystrophic subjects
may be degenerative rather than primary, but no
abnormal chemical product has yet been detected in
the tissues of patients with any of the conditions here
spoken of as tissue defects.

It is highly probable that chemical defects, or errors of
metabolism, are very common, although any individual
error is rarely met with. Those which we know proclaim
their presence in some obvious way, or are detected
because they respond to often applied tests. Others
which do not so advertise themselves may readily escape
notice. For example, if the copper tests for detection of
glucose were not in daily use in medical work, there is
no symptom yet known by which the existence of that
rare anomaly pentosuria could have been detected.

Presumably some chemical mutations are beneficial
or at least harmless; but some render their subjects
liable to morbid developments of particular kinds. To
the victim of congenital porphyria light behaves as a
poison, the cystinuric is always in danger of calculous
troubles, and the alcaptonuric is wont to develop in late
life an osteo-arthritis of characteristic kind and distribution. By the study of such anomalies one seems to
approach very nearly the solution of some cases of morbid predisposition.

When we turn to the consideration of the infective
maladies we find ourselves confronted by a new set of

problems, and problems of the greatest importance because such maladies are responsible for the great bulk of
human sickness, and take the heaviest toll of human life.
In them the organism is called upon to wage an active
fight against highly trained external enemies, whether
bacteria, viruses, or protozoa, and the signs and symptoms which compose the pictures of such diseases are
the evidences of that struggle.

Even against chemical poisons taken by mouth, or by
other channels, there are some means of defence. Every
active drug is a poison, when taken in large enough
doses; and in some subjects a dose* which is innocuous
to the majority of people has toxic effects, whereas
others show exceptional tolerance of the same drug.

Some chemical poisons are destroyed in the tissues,
provided that the dose given be not too large, and others
are combined up with substances to hand, and so
rendered innocuous and got rid of.

Against bacterial invaders more subtle protective
mechanisms have been evolved, some to destroy the invaders and others to render their toxins innocuous. The
protective substances present in the blood and tissues,
antitoxins, agglutinins, opsonins and the like, are undoubtedly chemical compounds, but as yet we know
nothing of them save the properties from which they
derive their names. When an invasion occurs the
specific antibody is formed, if not already present, and
an immunity is acquired which lasts for weeks, months,
years, or even for the remainder of life.

* *a dose* This is a statement of what is now sometimes called 'pharmacogenetics'. But, as always, Garrod points out that distributions have two
extremes. An ordinary dose of a drug may be toxic to some, but it is also
useless to others. That could represent a handicap too.

Apart from this natural process, the appropriate antibodies may be administered in the serum of an immunized animal, or their formation may be stimulated by a vaccine containing the toxin.

This, as was pointed out in an earlier section, greatly aggravates the difficulty of determining how far a natural immunity against infective diseases exists; for so many individuals have acquired immunity in one or other of these ways or even by exposure to contagion apart from any actual attack of the disease under investigation.

The clinical evidence of the existence of natural immunity, and also of unusual liability to particular maladies, is very strong, and is based upon the experience of many generations of medical men. It receives support from the results of statistical investigations of liability to tuberculosis for example, and from the results of the Schick test of liability to diphtheria. Yet such testimony gives a somewhat restrained answer. There is, moreover, testimony of clinical experience to the hereditary character of such immunities and liabilities.

Lastly, the so-called idiosyncrasies, disturbances of health out of all proportion to the external causes which provoke them, display the protest of the organism against the intrusion of some foreign substance, sometimes a drug, more often a foreign protein. It is not clear how far the phenomena observed in such cases have a protective purpose, as those of inflammation have; nor that the base histamine which plays a leading role in the production of the allergic syndrome is secreted by the damaged cells, rather than leaks from them when they are damaged.

But allergy is, to all appearance, a chemical event, and the highly specialized effects of particular exciting substances, the pollen of a special plant or the exhalation of an animal of a particular species, point to a large personal element in connexion with such phenomena. Moreover, we can hardly doubt that in many, if not in all cases, the susceptibility is inborn. Such idiosyncrasies are apt to occur in several members of a family, but the exciting cause is not always the same in the different members of a family. In the grave diseases which pertain to the allergic group, such as asthma in some at least of its forms, and angioneurotic oedema which, when it affects the larynx, may cause death by suffocation, the hereditary factor is often strongly marked.

It might be claimed that what used to be spoken of as a diathesis is nothing else but chemical individuality.[*] But to our chemical individualities are due our chemical *merits* as well as our chemical shortcomings; and it is more nearly true to say that the factors which confer upon us our predispositions to, and immunities from the various mishaps which are spoken of as diseases, are inherent in our very chemical structure; and even in the molecular groupings which confer upon us our individualities, and which went to the making of the chromosomes from which we sprang.

* *It might be claimed* . . .The first sentence is the leitmotiv of *Inborn factors in disease*. Garrod's final paragraph has a tone similar to that of Darwin's last in *Origin of species*.

INDEX

Abiotrophies, or tissue defects, 82–96, 153.
Achlorhydria, constitutional, 81,121.
Albinism, 64, 120.
Alcaptonuria, 112.
Allergic diseases, 34, 143.
— idiosyncrasies, 135 et seq., 157.
Anaphylaxis, 135, 139.
Angioneurotic oedema, 34, 137, 143, 157.
Arthritic diathesis, arthritism, 15.
— —, Bouchard's theory of, 16.
Asthma, 34, 143, 157.
Atavism, 61, 66.

Bacteria, evolution of, 59.
Blood corpuscles, red, in haemolytic jaundice, 87.
Blood groups, 43.
— —, inheritance of, 44.
— —, racial distribution of, 44.
— —, in twins, 68.
Bones, fragility of, with blue sclerotics, 84–5.
— —, in osteosclerosis, 85.
— —, otosclerosis with, 85.

Chemical individuality, 39–52.
— mutations, 41, 100, 154.
— anomalies, 100.
Chromosomes and individuality, 40, 148, 157.
Consanguinity of parents, in connexion with heredity, 65.
Constitution, 20 et passim.
Constitutional clinics, 19, 75.
Cystinuria, 102.
— and calculus formation, 104.

Deficiency diseases, 32, 150.
— —, predisposition to, 33.

Dermatography, 137.
Diabetes, in twins, 72.
Diatheses, the doctrine of, 9–24.
—, definitions of, 11, 12, 13, 18.
Diphtheria and the Schick test, 129.
Disease and health, 25–39.
—, definitions of, 26.
—, evolution and, 52–60.
—, heredity of, 60–73.
—, relation of to physical structure, 22, 74–81.
—, acquired in utero, 61.
Drugs, idiosyncrasies with regard to, 143.
Dystrophia myotonica, 93.

Ectoderm, defect of, 83.
Endocrine glands, syndromes due to diseases of, 35.
— —, influence of, on bodily form, 50.
Environment, influence of, in family diseases, 63.
Erect posture, diseases due to, 49.
Ergosterol, vitamin D formed by irradiation of, 33, 116.
Errors of metabolism, diseases due to, 96–122.
Evolution and disease, 52–60.
— of infective agents, 53, 59.
— of protective mechanisms, 58, 127.

Finger prints of twins, 68.
Form, bodily, in relation to disease, 74–81.

Gastric hypertonus, 80.
Gastroptosis, 80.
Gaucher's disease, 89–91.
— —, part played by kerasin in, 90.

PRINTED IN GREAT BRITAIN AT THE UNIVERSITY PRESS, OXFORD
BY JOHN JOHNSON, PRINTER TO THE UNIVERSITY

EPILOGUE: GENETIC PREDISPOSITION AFTER GARROD

Diathesis is nothing else but chemical individuality. (The inborn factors in disease, p. 157)

With characteristic elegance and understatement, Garrod advanced a view of medicine in *The inborn factors in disease* that was much at variance with the one prevailing in his time. At its centre are the inborn errors, biochemical aberrations due to hereditary abnormalities of enzymes. These abnormalities, he reasoned, must be exemplary of other hereditary differences, also in their origins chemical, but expressed sometimes in other forms such as anatomical anomalies. These differences need not be abnormal; indeed most must be normal and must underlie all the variation we see among human beings. Each person has his quota of such qualities inherited through parents from distant antecedents and expressed as a chemical individuality. These hereditary differences represent the wherewithal of evolution; they are tested in life and represent, in relation to the environment, a person's strengths and weaknesses. If the latter, they are inborn predispositions to disease, or diatheses, emerging as overt disease only in the face of such provocations as micro-organisms, drugs, toxic substances even the wear and tear of ordinary life. So Garrod proposed that the causes of disease lie partly internally in a person's singular endowment, and partly in aspects of the environment for which that singularity is unsuited. It is not that either the individuality or the experiences are of themselves harmful, rather disease is a consequence of their incongruence. So, if one were to try to summarize Garrod's perception in a sentence, it might be that the interactions of human beings with nature are strongly conditioned by human history, both biological and cultural, and disease is a consequence of a mismatch between individual versions of these two historical currents.

We cannot expect Garrod to have anticipated in any detail how

[185]

we conceive of disease today; the question is whether his line of reasoning is in any way predictive of and relevant to current views; and whether the history he was a part of and in part made concerns us now. In fact, it seems that his speculations are representative of emerging concepts of health and disease in which individuality is increasingly accepted as playing a part. Molecular genetics has made a reality of chemical individuality, and in a form that falls readily into Garrod's context. The remainder of this epilogue will be devoted to observing how well Garrod's ideas stand up in the light of modern knowledge and to examining what impact a modern version of chemical individuality is having on medical investigation and practice.

CONTEXTS

If the basic question in medicine is 'why does this patient have this disease now?', it is not a new one; it, or one like it, was posed by Caleb Parry in the 18th century and by King (1982) and Rose (1985) for example, in our own times. Answers to the question, which are the solutions to the medical problem at hand, are changing constantly as medical knowledge and fashions change. But the question and the nature of the problem it addresses do not change because there is always need for diagnosis of the disease which affects the patient, to understand the pathogenesis of the disease's manifestations, and to explain the events that started it.

Knowledge of the cause and the pathogenesis of a disease are antecedents to its treatment and, perhaps, for its avoidance or prevention. Medicine, as it tends to be practised and taught, is concerned more with manifestations and pathogenesis than with cause. This may explain why a reviewer (Watkins 1986) of the *Oxford companion to medicine*—which was published in 1986—was not vastly enchanted by its contents. He thought the *Companion*, excellent as it was, revealed all too clearly that medicine—the discipline—has no intellectual content analogous to that of quantum mechanics, for example. Medicine, he opined, is an

[186]

assemblage of facts, near-facts, and anecdotes upon which the physician draws for diagnosis and treatment of the patient's disease. One way to make a case against this indictment of medicine, is to adopt Garrod's point of view about disease: that there is often a genetic predisposition to it. Such a view of the cause of a disease anticipates its consequences; avoidance or prevention of disease may follow.

Garrod's major contribution to medicine did, in fact, begin with an anecdote—stained diapers or urine that blackened on exposure to air. But he proceeded to identify an important fact, namely that an excess of homogentisic acid in the urine explained the anecdote. He considered the homogentisic aciduria to be a form of chemical individuality. He proposed that it was inherited according to recognizable laws of biology. From such anecdotes and facts Garrod went on to create an hypothesis of enduring intellectual interest which he articulated in the Croonian Lectures to the Royal Society in 1908 and in the corresponding version in book form, his *Inborn errors of metabolism* published in 1909 and further expanded in the 1923 edition.

In his second book *The inborn factors in disease*, Garrod expands his concept of individuality to say that it is predisposition to disease. This point of view has become clear and relevant in at least three contexts of medicine: first, the knowledge base upon which medicine operates; second, the changing character of disease; and third, medical education and its counterpart—medical care.

KNOWLEDGE

Garrod understood the nature–nurture theme. He knew that an encounter which overwhelmed health was an important cause of disease in his day. But his awareness of chemical individuality led him to believe that human singularity could in itself constitute a predisposition to disease whether the encounter was universal or particular. Garrod observed (p. 149, *Inborn factors*) that 'man has to struggle against his own individual short-comings upon the one hand and against physical agents, chemicals, poisons and the attacks of pathogenic organisms on the other hand'. The practical challenge was, then as it is now, to identify the cause of the individual shortcomings and to deal with them. As long as they were abstractions, they could not be approached and they could not command the interest Garrod believed they deserved. New knowledge has affirmed the correctness of Garrod's vision of human individuality; more important, it helps us to anticipate genetic predisposition and to prevent or avoid its associated disease. In this sense, the intellectual content of medicine derived from genetics contributes to the social dimensions of medicine if it influences practice and benefits the patient.

Garrod used the tools of biochemistry to measure human chemical individuality at the metabolite level. His successors found the corresponding evidence at the polypeptide level. From these phenotypes came the inference that human individuality could be found at the level of chromosomes and genes, when the latter became accessible to analysis. Advances in cytogenetics revealed the correct number of chromosomes in man about 20 years after Garrod's death. Soon thereafter came the first evidence that the cause of a human disease (Down syndrome) could be seen at the chromosome level. The explosive growth of knowledge about DNA and the nature of genes, which occurred while the cytogeneticists were expanding their knowledge, set the scene for the emergence of techniques to study human genes at the molecular level.

Knowledge also grew with the discovery of genetic polymorphisms, a form of chemical individuality that Garrod anticipated but did not witness in its full display. The first evidence appeared in Garrod's own lifetime with Landsteiner's discovery of ABO blood groups. Then in the 1950s, when electrophoresis was invented, the evidence for polymorphisms in blood proteins appeared. This was followed by the delineation of extraordinary variation between individuals in human leucocyte antigens (HLA polymorphism). Perhaps we would have expected to find polymorphism on surfaces of cells and in proteins of extracellular fluids where the agents of the environment are encountered but now it is apparent that polymorphism reaches right into the interior of cells to affect soluble cellular proteins.

As a form of chemical individuality such polymorphisms are a generalized phenomenon found throughout the phyla, orders, and species (Harris 1980; Lewontin 1985). In general, they are neutral to selection, meaning they confer no apparent advantage or cost. However, that holds only for the universal experience shared by the species; under a particular circumstance these polymorphisms might be advantageous or deleterious. It is this feature that attracts medical attention, and Garrod, ever percep- tive, speculated that chemical individuality could confer either resistance or susceptibility to an agent of disease. How right he was. Whereas we find that much genetic variation is harmful, we also find that the compensating advantage of polymorphisms such as sickle haemoglobin and the thalassaemias explains why they occur at such high frequencies in certain populations, notably those that were historically exposed to malaria. J. B. S. Haldane, a young man in Garrod's years as Regius Professor of Physic at Oxford, was to propose not long after Garrod had died that selection was the mechanism which had driven these particu- lar polymorphisms to their high frequencies in modern popula- tions and that their compensating advantage against malaria infection was conferred by the chemical individuality of haemo- globin.

Polymorphic phenotypes originate, of course, in genotypes. However, the extent of polymorphism in DNA greatly exceeds that which we would have predicted from phenotype, and it is what Garrod might have called the ultimate chemical individu- ality. Selection can act only on phenotypes but the objects selected are those parts of the genome which regulate or are translated into phenotype (Sober 1984). Sequences of nucleotides occur in human DNA which are not translated into phenotype; indeed they comprise the largest part of the genome. Accordingly, they can evolve by mutation more freely. The great diversity of DNA between individuals, particularly in their non-transcribing sequences, was discovered when molecular genetic methods made it possible to analyse the nucleotide sequences of translated (exons) and non-translated DNA. The interindividual diversity is enormous and the fact of it heightens the interest in how human genomes will be sequences when that project is undertaken. Two forms of DNA polymorphism have attracted particular notice. One concerns so-called hypervariable regions which contain variable numbers of tandem repeats (VNTRs) that are unique to individuals and are being used for legal and forensic purposes (Jeffreys *et al.* 1985). The other is the restriction fragment length polymorphism (RFLP), the product of recognition sites where a specific endonuclease (restriction enzyme) cuts double-strand DNA into fragments of characteristic length. Change (mutation) in the nucleotide sequence at a restriction site changes the length of the DNA fragment obtained by digesting DNA with the appropriate endonuclease. When particular VNTRs and RFLPs in or near genes of medical interest are associated with occurrence of disease in those who inherit the gene, the former can serve as 'markers' of predisposition. Here then is the ultimate form of chemical individuality and it can be recruited for medical purposes.

VNTRs and RFLPs are being used to develop genetic and physical maps of the human genome and the makers of the maps can capitalize on one of Garrod's own early findings. He recognized that an unusually high proportion of his patients with alcaptonuria were offspring of consanguineous marriages. Accordingly, they were likely to be genetically homozygous for the mutant gene they had inherited. A modern strategy for mapping genes that cause disease uses consanguinity to find adjacent regions of DNA that are homozygous by descent and recognizable through previously mapped RFLPs and VNTRs (Lander and Botstein 1987).

Three broad classics of genetic disease will eventually be accommodated by the chromosome atlases we already have and the genome maps under development; chromosomal aberrations; Mendelian (single-gene) disorders; and multifactorial diseases. This categorization is useful only in that it tells something about the salience of the genetic component as a cause of disease (Denniston 1982; Matsunaga 1982). Chromosomal disorders involving the number or structure of chromosomes are largely diseases of embryogenesis and morphogenesis. Accordingly, they are disorders whose expression has occurred in a universal human environment—the womb. Chromosomal disorders are very frequent, affecting perhaps 70 per cent or more of implantations, and 50 per cent of recognized abortions. Viability selection on the associated phenotypes is great; less than 1 per cent of individuals with this form of disease are live-born and most of the latter die early in postnatal life. Down syndrome (trisomy 21) is the major form of surviving chromosomal disease.

Mendelian phenotypes are apparently less prevalent, by comparison with chromosomal disorders. More than 4400 Mendelian phenotypes are known (McKusick 1988) of which about three-quarters are diseases. In the aggregate these diseases affect at least 1 per cent of live-born humans. They make their presence known, in 90 per cent of the associated phenotypes, before puberty—most of the remainder in early adult life (Costa *et al.* 1985). In general, the earlier the onset the more severe their effect and the more likely the life-span of an affected individual will be shortened. This class of genetic disease is expressed for the most part regardless of experience and extraordinary measures are required for its treatment; the remainder of the Mendelian diseases are phenotypes expressed in particular environments, which, if avoided, will avert occurrence of disease.

In the third class, so-called multifactorial disease, mutation and encounter are both necessary components of cause; neither alone is sufficient to cause the disease. Multifactorial disease is the most prevalent form of 'genetic' disease—affecting up to 60 per cent of long-living persons in one recent estimate (Baird *et al.* 1988).

This classification, broad as it is and useful as it now may be for some purposes, is too categorical for ours because it implies that diseases are either genetic or not genetic. To use that taxonomy undermines Garrod's (and our) concept of diathesis. Accordingly, we should study some examples which are exemplary of Garrod's ideas; they are: familial hypercholesterolaemia, phenylketonuria, and Hartnup disorder. Each reveals the chemical individuality which Garrod considered to lie at the root of

diathesis. Although each disease has an ultimate cause in mutation, it also has a proximate cause in the experience of the patient,
just as the evolutionary process has ultimate and proximate causes
(Mayr 1961). Each also illustrates another theme, latent in Garrod's work but one he did articulate, that recognition of chemical
individuality can be used to prevent the disease. They illustrate
very well how works of science bear upon the practice of medicine.

THREE EXAMPLES OF DIATHESIS

Familial hypercholesterolaemia

In 1910, James B. Herrick gave a paper entitled 'Certain clinical
features of sudden obstruction of the coronary arteries' at the
annual meeting of the Association of American Physicians.
Recalling the occasion many years later, Herrick remembered
being both elated at offering a substantial contribution and
deflated by its reception. In his words, the paper 'fell flat as a
pancake' (Harvey 1986). When asked about this episode Paul D.
White said 'Herrick's classical paper on coronary thrombosis was
before my time, but I wonder if I would have taken it in any more
than did Herrick's colleagues, who apparently missed its significance for nearly a decade even though they heard him present it'.
In 1985, 75 years after Herrick's presentation, Michael S. Brown
and Joseph L. Goldstein received both universal applause and the
Nobel Prize for having discovered an explanation of Herrick's
observations (Brown and Goldstein 1986).

Between 1910 and 1985, Garrod had given his lectures,
produced the second edition of *Inborn errors*, and written and
published *Inborn factors in disease*; others had accepted Herrick's
observation and gone on to recognize atherosclerosis and
coronary artery disease as major causes of premature death in
adulthood in Western populations; yet others had assigned to our
style of living and its associated risk factors the principal causes
of coronary artery disease. Only in the last 20 years of the 75 did
genetic determinants of coronary artery disease receive any

serious attention. None the less, the belated awareness of familial predisposition to coronary artery disease, and the emergence of evidence for Mendelian forms of it, has provided a much clearer understanding of the clinical manifestations, pathogenesis and causes of this disease. One form of coronary artery disease, the condition now known as familial hypercholesterolaemia (FH) has attracted particular notice. FH is an inborn error of metabolism, it is among the most frequent affecting humans and it is one of the first to be well understood at the levels of cause, pathogenesis, and manifestations of its specific phenotype. Its importance in medicine is not in doubt.

Cholesterol is an essential metabolite. It is required as a constituent of the plasma membrane of all cells in the human body and it is a precursor of steroid hormones and bile acids. When not provided by diet, it is made by the body. The balance between nurture (diet) and nature (synthesis) is regulated and thereby cholesterol homeostasis is achieved. One aspect of Brown and Goldstein's achievement was their evidence that a receptor on the surface of cells is a principal component of cholesterol homeostasis. The receptor molecule is coded for by a gene on chromosome 19. All known mutations at this locus impair function of the receptor and disrupt cholesterol homeostasis by blocking uptake of packaged cholesterol (the low-density lipoprotein–cholesterol particle). The block in cholesterol traffic is analogous to the block in metabolic pathways envisaged by Garrod. Heterozygotes have about twofold elevation of plasma total cholesterol (350–550 mg/dl); their number is estimated to be about 1 in 500 in Western populations. The rarer homozygous phenotype (plasma cholesterol 650–1000 mg/dl, incidence about 1 per million births) is determined by inheritance of two mutant genes at the receptor locus. A gene dosage effect is apparent in FH; the homozygous phenotype is more severe, occurs earlier, and is harder to treat than the heterozygous phenotype. From the knowledge that receptor deficiency explains the disease came proposals for early diagnosis and treatment to prevent it.

Herrick's contribution was to propose that obstruction of

coronary blood flow was a cause of myocardial infarction and death in mankind. Studies followed exposing various risk factors, both constitutional and environmental, such as sex, body weight, work habits, blood pressure, diet, smoking, and alcohol consumption, each contributing to the pathogenesis of coronary artery disease; still the tendency was to think typologically, to consider coronary artery disease as a single disease. Then, in 1973, Goldstein and colleagues (1973*a*, *b*) showed that a third of the survivors of myocardial infarctions under the age of 60 had single-gene, dominantly inherited disorders of lipid homeostasis; one of these was familial hypercholesterolaemia. One had now to believe that coronary artery disease was many diseases, genetic predisposition playing a different role in the different forms.

Treatment of FH requires two approaches: one to reduce the overburden of cholesterol, the other to suppress overproduction. Dietary restriction is not sufficient because it is offset by up-regulation of cholesterol synthesis in the cell. There are two agents for treatment. Non-absorbable bile-acid binding resins, taken by mouth, increase the fractional catabolic rate for LDL cholesterol. Mevinolin and like drugs (e.g. lovostatin and compactin) suppress cholesterol synthesis and do not need the receptor to penetrate the cell. Together, the binding resin and the inhibitor restore near-normal cholesterol homeostasis in the heterozygous phenotype. It is anticipated that early treatment will significantly improve prognosis of heterozygotes.

The LDL receptor has been isolated and characterized. It has 839 amino acids and five domains which, beginning at the NH-terminus, are: a cholesterol-ligand binding domain (292 amino acids), a domain (about 400 amino acids) mimicking the epidermal growth factor (EGF) precursor; a domain (58 amino acids) rich in O-linked sugars; a trans-membrane domain (of 22–25 hydrophobic amino acids) permitting insertion of the receptor into the plasma membrane; and a cytoplasmic domain (50 amino acids) necessary for targeting the receptor to coated pits in the plasma membrane.

The corresponding gene spans approximately 45 kilobases of DNA. The gene is divided into 18 exons (coding sequences) and

17 introns (intervening sequences). Structural domains in the protein correlate well with exon sequences in the gene. The signal sequence is encoded by the first exon at the 5' end of the gene. The cholesterol-ligand binding domain is encoded by an adjacent series of exons moving toward the 3' end of the gene. The EGF precursor domain comprises eight exons in the middle of the gene, which have strong homologies with the exons encoding EGF precursor itself (an apparent example of an information 'cassette' being duplicated and used for multiple purposes during evolution). The O-linked sugar domain is encoded by a single exon. Two pairs of exons encode the membrane-spanning and the cytoplasmic domains respectively. The last exon at the 3' end of the gene encodes 12 amino acids at the COOH terminus of the cytoplasmic domain and 2.5 kilobases of untranslated nucleotides.

Many mutations affecting the FH gene have been identified (Fig. 1). They comprise insertions and deletions of DNA segments, nonsense and missense point mutations; they affect all

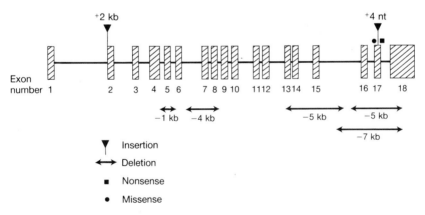

FIG. 1. An example of chemical individuality at the DNA level. The diagram shows a variety of mutations in the LDL receptor gene which is about 45 kilobases long with 18 exons and 17 introns. Each mutation was found in a different family. Each is expressed as a different form of deficient receptor activity (from Brown and Goldstein 1986).

exons except some encoding part of the EGF-precursor domain. Accordingly, familial hypercholesterolaemia due to LDL receptor deficiency, which is only one form of coronary artery disease, itself has many causes.

Each mutant genotype has its own polypeptide phenotype; it follows that the associated clinical FH phenotypes should be heterogeneous even if the mutations that cause them are at one locus. Heterogeneity of clinical manifestations in the FH phenotype is a clinical fact. That its cause may lie in genetic heterogeneity is a reasonable hypothesis. But it cannot be the sole explanation. Among French Canadians, two-thirds of FH heterozygotes have the same mutation; it is a null allele with a 10-kilobase deletion at the 5′ end of the gene (Hobbs *et al.* 1987), and a founder effect probably explains its ubiquity in the French Canadian population. None the less, persons with this particular mutation (in its heterozygous or homozygous form) show great individuality in severity of the associated disease. We do not know yet why this is the case but it implies that other genes and experiences must also influence the FH phenotype; it might be possible, among French Canadian probands at least, to identify those other components. And of special clinical relevance, with a single molecular probe it will be possible to diagnose the specific genetic predisposition and to initiate treatment early in the majority of French Canadians at risk for FH disease.

The example of familial hypercholesterolaemia is useful here for several reasons. First, it is a superb illustration of chemical individuality. Second, it shows how modern molecular methods can reveal the origins of individuality; in this case they are the mutations in a gene encoding an arbiter of cholesterol homeostasis. Third, it reveals how knowledge of pathogenesis (here it is dishomeostasis of cholesterol metabolism) points to a potentially effective treatment of its consequences (and in this case, the accelerated atherogenesis). Last, it indicates how physicians may be able to use this knowledge to anticipate and prevent disease in those who are relatives of an affected patient and, if they inherited the mutation segregating in their family, are at risk for premature onset of coronary artery disease.

[196]

GENETIC PREDISPOSITION AFTER GARROD

Phenylketonuria (PKU)

PKU is a cause of mental retardation (Scriver and Clow 1980). It was first recognized as an entity in 1934 (Fölling). The chemical manifestations of PKU derive from an overburden of phenylalanine in body fluids and overproduction of its metabolic derivatives. The name of the condition recognizes its principal metabolite phenylpyruvic acid—the keto acid product of transaminated phenylalanine. About three-quarters of the phenylalanine molecules in human metabolism should normally enter a catabolic pathway that yields CO_2 and H_2O; conversion of phenylalanine to tyrosine is the first step in the pathway. The hydroxylation reaction forming tyrosine is catalysed by the enzyme phenylalanine hydroxylase and the homozygous PKU phenotype has a severe deficiency of phenylalanine hydroxylase activity. Deficient activity causes the substrate phenylalanine to accumulate and divert into pathways, otherwise minor now hyperactive, to form unusual metabolites in unusual amounts, such as phenylpyruvic acid.

Four important facts about PKU were known by the early 1950s. It was a Mendelian disorder and the disease phenotype was inherited as an autosomal recessive. Deficient activity of a single enzyme explained the chemical findings. The chemical findings were almost uniformly accompanied by disease (mental retardation). The principal chemical finding (accumulation of phenylalanine) involved an amino acid that could not be synthesized by the body and was thus an essential nutrient; that is to say, an experience (dietary phenylalanine) as well as a mutation were both necessary causes of the disease.

Two further facts were then reported. First, the intake of the essential nutrient (phenylalanine) could be controlled through dietary means and the overburden of phenylalanine and its derivatives reduced. Second, there was at birth no overburden of phenylalanine and no evidence of mental retardation in the PKU homozygote. The occurrence of mental retardation was dependent on the development of persistent, severe postnatal hyperphenylalaninaemia. Accordingly, early diagnosis of the PKU phenotype and early treatment of it with a low-phenylalanine diet might prevent the disease manifestations of PKU. This point of view has subsequently been proven correct, by and large, in programmes where newborn screening and treatment of PKU were implemented. Such programmes are now part of health care systems in most countries of the developed world.

The inherited causes of impaired phenylalanine hydroxylation involve several loci in the human genome because there are several components in the hydroxylation reaction, each dependent on a specific polypeptide. They are the phenylalanine hydroxylase apoenzyme, the enzymes responsible for synthesis of its tetrahydrobiopterin cofactor, and dihydrobiopterin reductase which maintains the cofactor in reduced form. The gene for the phenylalanine hydroxylase polypeptide has been mapped to a locus on the long arm of chromosome 12; it has been sequenced, and several mutations responsible for classical PKU have been characterized. Dihydropteridine reductase maps to chromosome 4 and the gene has been cloned. The genes controlling synthesis of tetrahydrobiopterin are not yet mapped; several steps are required for cofactor biosynthesis. From this we learn that the chemical individuality recognizable as hyperphenylalaninaemia could have many genetic forms caused by mutations in several genes.

Chemical individuality at the human phenylalanine hydroxylase locus has been revealed (DiLella and Woo 1987) in a manner that would no doubt have delighted Garrod. The chromosomes on which alleles occur and cause hyperphenylalaninaemia were characterized using a full-length human cDNA probe. Restriction enzymes identify nine highly polymorphic DNA segments (RFLPs) at the phenylalanine hydroxylase locus. The pattern of RFLPs on a particular chromosome constitutes a haplotype; over a thousand different haplotypes could exist with these polymorphic restriction sites. A study of Danish individuals among whom the PKU phenotype is prevalent showed that only 12 haplotypes occurred and about 90 per cent of the PKU alleles were associated with only four haplotypes. Moreover, specific mutant alleles tended to be associated with particular haplotypes in this population. For example, a G to A transition at the 5′ donor splice site of intron 12 causes aberrant RNA splicing and skips exon 12 in the mature RNA. An unstable truncated polypeptide is produced. This mutation associates with haplotype 3 and it causes the PKU phenotype. Another PKU mutation involves a C to T transition in exon 12 with substitution of tryptophan for arginine at residue 408 of the polypeptide. The mutant enzyme is inactive. This mutation associates with haplotype 2. The tendency of alleles to associate with haplotypes is of clinical interest. Probands homozygous for haplotypes 2 and 3 in the Danish population have the PKU phenotype whereas probands with haplotypes 1 and 4 usually have a less severe hyperphenylalaninaemic phenotype (non-PKU) without mental retardation in the untreated state; the mutant alleles associated with haplotypes 1 and 4 have not yet been characterized.

We now know the following: hyperphenylalaninaemia is a phenotype caused by mutations in one of several genes; PKU is one form of hyperphenylalaninaemia; PKU is itself a heterogenous disease because it has multiple causes (alleles) at the hydroxylase locus. Accordingly hyperphenylalaninaemia and PKU are analogous to coronary artery disease and receptor-deficient familial hypercholesterol and there are similar implications for treatment, prognosis, and counselling of probands with hyperphenylalaninaemia.

How does PKU illustrate Garrod's particular concept of diathesis and how has the fact of genetic predisposition in this disease been used? First, PKU (and its variants) is a diathesis because its harm is provoked by an experience (phenylalanine in the diet), yet the experience is harmful only to those genetically predisposed. Second, knowledge of the associated chemical individuality has been used to prevent the disease. Universal newborn screening to detect hyperphenylalaninaemia can, through early diagnosis and treatment, prevent disease in nearly every affected case born into a population. Moreover, screening for chemical individuality (Fig. 2) is clearly a more efficient means to prevent the disease than counselling families after occurrence of the first case.

[199]

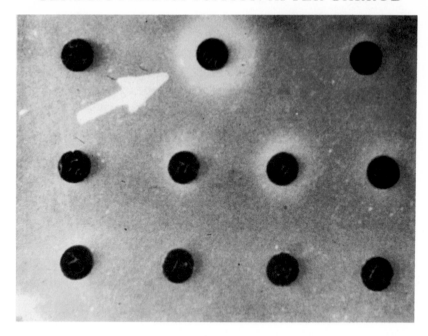

FIG. 2. An example of a chemical individuality, in this case at the metabolite level. The photograph shows a Guthrie plate of agar containing bacterial spores and an inhibitor of their growth. The black circles are filter paper discs impregnated with blood, one disc per newborn infant. A disc which contains an abnormally elevated concentration of phenylalanine will cause the amino acid to diffuse into the agar, offset the inhibitor effect, and allow the bacteria to multiply. A growth zone (white ring) indicates hyperphenylalaninaemia in the blood sample. The width of the ring is proportional to the concentration of phenylalanine in the disc. The Guthrie test is used in newborn screening programmes for early detection of infants with phenylketonuria and other forms of hyperphenylalaninaemia.

The PKU story is not yet complete. There is evidence that early diagnosis and treatment are not quite a panacea for PKU disease because they do not eliminate its consequences in every patient. Treated patients with classical PKU, as a group, have small but significant IQ deficits and some individuals have poor outcomes despite apparently good treatment. Why this is the case is not yet known—it may relate to the genetic heterogeneity of the condition—but it does introduce a note of uncertainty where, formerly, confidence was high that this is a fully treatable genetic disease. Accordingly parents who have learned that they are at risk for having a PKU offspring may want to avoid altogether the costs—however small—of that genotype. In other words, they must deal with genetic predisposition to a disease. The majority of such couples could now receive reproductive counselling based on ascertainment of the fetal genotype by molecular genetic methods. Whereas there are no data to reveal how parents might behave, given this option, the situation illustrates again the relevance of Garrod's ideas. Molecular analysis of DNA at the PKU locus can identify the chemical individuality that constitutes genetic predisposition to a disease. Some families will use that opportunity to avoid possible occurrence of disease. The approach is not necessarily worse or better than newborn screening, only different. Both approaches capitalize on the phenomena of chemical individuality and genetic predisposition espoused by Garrod.

Hartnup disorder versus Hartnup disease

This condition also illustrates Garrod's concept of diathesis and it highlights the importance of the question: why does this patient have this disease, now?

Hartnup disorder takes its name from its first patient (Baron *et al.* 1956; Jepson 1978). As a young man he developed dermatitis and neurological manifestations following exposure to sunlight at levels exceptional for him. His self-limited disease was noted to have features reminiscent of pellagra. Investigations revealed he had a recessively inherited impairment of amino acid transport, expressed in kidney and intestine. A large group of neutral-charge amino acids was affected; it included tryptophan and five other essential amino acids (threonine, valine, isoleucine, leucine, phenylalanine) and five non-essential amino acids. Following the first report in 1953 of 'Hartnup disease'—as it was then called—

there were others, each describing patients with the abnormal membrane transport phenotype and an associated disease—'pellagra-like' in some, impaired psychomotor development in others. These additional reports seemed to support the opinion that the homozygous Hartnup phenotype was a disease. Most reviews of the topic perpetuated this point of view.

The discovery of 'Hartnup disease' was facilitated by access to a new and simple laboratory method, namely two-dimensional partition chromatography of amino acids on filter paper. The chemical individuality of the Hartnup subject was instantly recognizable by the characteristic pattern of urine amino acids on the filter paper chromatogram. One could recognize the pattern the way one knew a face. About a decade after the Hartnup discovery, the chromatographic method was modified for mass screening of newborn urine samples. As a result, dozens of infants with the Hartnup urine amino acid pattern were detected wherever newborn urine screening was practised. Most of these cases never showed any evidence of disease during later life. It then became the convention, on the basis of the prospective experience, to say that Hartnup 'disease' was not a disease and to counsel accordingly. This tactic left an important fact in limbo; it was not apparent why so many retrospectively ascertained cases had presented with disease, whereas the screened cases developed none.

A conventional explanation for the occurrence of disease in retrospectively diagnosed Hartnup cases is bias of ascertainment; cases are diagnosed because they have an incidental disease which brings them to notice. One cannot say whether the disease has anything to do with the gene and one has no idea how many with the gene might have the disease. A prospective study avoids the bias. A prospective study of Hartnup cases was eventually done about a quarter century after the condition was first reported (Scriver *et al.* 1987).

Twenty-one subjects aged from 1 to 29 years, with a confirmed homozygous Hartnup phenotype and all diagnosed by newborn screening, were evaluated and compared with 19 unaffected siblings. With only two exceptions, the Hartnup subjects and their sibs were found to be normal and similar in somatic growth, intellectual development, school performance, and medical history. The exceptions were a Hartnup boy with delayed development and a Hartnup girl who developed a pellagra-like illness during treatment of a putative milk allergy; the treatment involved removal of cow's milk from the diet. The two symptomatic individuals were otherwise not different from the non-symptomatic Hartnup cases in the study. All evidence indicated they had the conventional Hartnup mutation. Yet one wants to know why these particular Hartnup cases had developed clinical manifestations, wheras 19 others did not. The answer appears to lie in the domain of diathesis.

The Hartnup gene product participates in a metabolic network which determines homeostasis of plasma amino acid values. In theory, mutation affecting the function of that gene and its product should impair plasma amino acid homeostasis. However, the Hartnup mutation does not have a significant effect on plasma amino homeostasis, at least in Hartnup subjects treated as a group. There is an explanation for this surprising finding.

Amino acid transport into and out of cells is so important and complex a function that it is not accommodated by a single genetic locus and its product. There are multiple amino acid carriers in tissues and one assumes there is a corresponding plethora of genes (none of the genes has yet been cloned or mapped in man). Mutation at the Hartnup locus is tolerated quite well—or so the evidence in Hartnup disorder implies—because other transport systems can accommodate the essential nutrients, otherwise transported by the Hartnup system.

Every gene is expressed against a background of other genes in the organism; this is as true of man as it is of any other species. Broad phenotypes, which we call here plasma amino acid homeostasis, are therefore polygenic. The various genes controlling transport, synthesis, and catabolism of amino acids, and thus their pool sizes, are all required for homeostasis. Interplay of the products of these loci sets the phenotype value for a particular amino acid. Within the public phenotype, which we think of as the 'normal' value (which has a mean and a distribution of values around the mean), there are subsets of values with distributions narrower than the public distribution; these subsets can be called private phenotypes; they belong to the individuals who comprise the population. Accordingly, there are two types of normal values: public and private.

If the circumstances in which the values are obtained are the same for all individuals in the population—that is, the experiences that might raise or lower the values are shared by all persons—it follows that an individual with a low outlier private value is likely to be different from one with a high outlier value because of differences in their genotypes at the loci contributing to the homeostatic (phenotype) value. In this sense, the outliers are said to have different chemical individualities, and the determinants of their individuality are polygenic.

The Hartnup gene, in its homozygous state, is expressed against the background of all other genes contributing to amino acid homeostasis in the individual. This is true for all Hartnup individuals. The two symptomatic Hartnup patients and their sibs, in the aforementioned study, were extreme low outliers for their plasma amino acid phenotype values (Fig. 3).

Does this information help to explain why the 'lower outlier' Hartnup cases had disease and other Hartnup subjects, who did not have this phenotype, did not have the disease? The answer is a qualified yes. The low outlier plasma amino acid values in the symptomatic Hartnup subjects cannot be attributed to a homozygous effect of the Hartnup gene because their unaffected sibs were also the low outliers in the control group. Accordingly, the symptomatic Hartnup case appears to be predisposed to disease by the private value for plasma amino acid homeostasis. In this sense, such a person has a diathesis; the background sets a threshold against which the Hartnup gene plays out its effects. Accordingly, knowledge of the private phenotype has predictive value; it anticipates which individuals in the subset of the population with the superimposed Hartnup phenotype are likely to develop disease.

Can one do anything with this information? Again the answer is a qualified yes. Although the major chemical phenotype in

GENETIC PREDISPOSITION AFTER GARROD

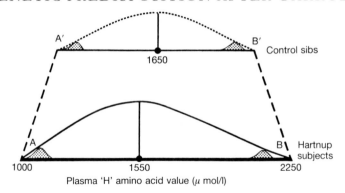

FIG. 3. An illustration of 'private' phenotypes in a population of phenotype values. The diagram shows frequency distributions of the summed values (moles/litre) for 10 amino acids in plasma of Hartnup subjects (front plane) and their sibs (near plane); the amino acids are those transported in the intestine and renal tubule on the carrier encoded by the Hartnup gene. The plasma value in a person is the phenotype value for expression of all genes encoding catalysts that determine the steady state. The means and distributions of phenotype values in Hartnup subjects and their sibs are not significantly different. However symptomatic Hartnup subjects (A) have low outlier values, implying that their genetic 'background' predisposes them to Hartnup disease under particular circumstances (e.g. reduction of diet protein intake). According to this view, high outlier Hartnup subjects (B) and low outlier sibs without the Hartnup phenotype (A') are not predisposed to disease.

Hartnup subjects is Mendelian, the associated disease is multifactorial in origin and occurs on a polygenic background. If only about 10 per cent of Hartnup probands are at risk for disease, and, if it is possible to predict who they are from their private polygenic phenotype, it follows that the high-risk persons should receive counselling to avoid experiences potentially harmful to them. Such persons should not have their protein intake reduced (as in the case of the child treated for milk allergy). Such persons apparently need supplements of the affected essential amino acids. Only continued observations will reveal whether this is a correct

[205]

view and whether it offers an effective way to prevent disease in the Hartnup case at elevated risk.

The Hartnup story shows us again how useful Garrod's theme of chemical individuality and diathesis can be when we try to understand human disease. Accordingly it is an interesting bridge to some thoughts about common multifactorial disease.

Conclusion

The three foregoing examples were used in a context of knowledge that has changed since Garrod's lifetime. They are now seen as distinctive entities yet they share a feature in common: at an earlier time each belonged to a larger class of disease in which its identity was blurred. These classes were coronary artery disease in the case of familial hypercholesterolaemia, mental retardation for phenylketonuria, and nutritional deficiency diseases—in particular pellagra—in the example of Hartnup disorder. If each disease belongs to a larger class, the former, by definition, is a particular cause of the latter; accordingly the latter, a superclass, must be multifactorial as to cause. In adopting Garrod's concept of chemical individuality, we have acquired a useful strategy for dealing with the superclass, the multifactorial entity; we divide it into subsets and deal with the latter, one by one. In our examples, it was a successful approach. It generated knowledge, led to preventive measures, and explained why a particular person developed a specific disease.

MULTIFACTORIAL DISEASES VIEWED AS DIATHESES

At the root of all three of the 'diatheses' described above are mutations at single loci; that is, in one sense, they are monogenic disorders and they are usually classified as such. Perhaps they would have been particularly congenial to Garrod *because* they are monogenic and are legitimately known as inborn errors. Most of the conditions he mentions in his book would now be known as inborn errors, but others such as gout, congenital malformation, allergies, and susceptibility to infection are likely now to be labelled multifactorial. In any case, he did not distinguish between Mendelian and multifactorial modes of inheritance. And in that, however unknowing, he was wise, since a categorical distinction between monogenic and multifactorial, however useful in diagnostic classification, makes no biological sense.

So, our three examples represent a sound basis on which to build models to explain other disorders of perhaps even more complex origin. For example, although the genetic contribution to multifactorial disorders is presumed to be multiple, it may turn out that only one or two genes, or at most a few, will account for many of the cases. It is a field which we enter with little to guide us beyond the idea of genetic susceptibility. But we do have good evidence that genes contribute in some way to many, indeed to most diseases. Hypertension, rheumatoid arthritis, diabetes, atherosclerosis and heart attack, gout, autoimmune diseases, peptic ulcers, senile dementia, psychotic behaviour, and several forms of cancer have all been demonstrated to be familial, and to show higher concordance between single-ovum twins than dizygotic pairs or non-twin sibs; for some, adoption studies have revealed the expected surplus of affected genetic as opposed to foster relatives. The nature of the genetic contribution to several of these diseases has been studied in both animals and man. Rats with several different forms of hypertension are known (cited in Childs 1983), rabbits with varying degree of resistance to infection have been bred by selection (Biozzi et al. 1984), and there are several strains of mice with autoimmune disease (McDevitt 1985). In man most of the autoimmune diseases have been shown to be associated with specific elements of the major histocompatibility complex (MHC), most frequently with type II alleles (Ryder et al. 1981). For example, type I diabetes is associated with DR3 and DR4, rheumatoid arthritis with DR4, systemic lupus with DR3, and so on. As for infections, more than 50 inborn errors of the immune system have been described; a recent one is a defect of monophosphate kinase 3, which raises markedly the risk for haemophilus influenzae B meningitis (Petersen et al. 1985). And the apparent virulence of microorganisms turns out to be more a property of biochemical and molecular congruence between organism and host than of the ability of the microbe to attack anyone it encounters (Childs *et al.* 1989). Perhaps chemical individuality is nowhere more easily demonstrated than in the mechanisms of defence that have evolved during millions of years of coexistence of man and microbe. Or, rather, as Garrod rightly pointed out (p. 124), we should say co-evolved since coexistence is possible only when both parties are capable of adapting. So the question, why does this person have this disease now, is going to turn out to be as readily answerable in regard to infections as to anything else, but in a way rather different from that which considers only the infective organism in the explanation of the subsequent disease.

Recombinant DNA methods, especially linkage analysis using gene fragments presumed to be genetically linked with genes involved in cause, promise much reward in the analysis of multifactorial disorders. Examples are: (1) RFLPs marking alleles specifying apolipoproteins A and B that represent apparent risk factors for coronary artery disease (Deeb *et al.* 1987; Goldbourt and Neufeld 1986); (2) a gene in chromosome 21 associated with some cases of Alzheimer's disease (Tanzi *et al.* 1987; St. George-Hyslop *et al.* 1987); and (3) genes on chromosomes 11 and the X that distinguish families with manic-depressive disorder (Egelund *et al.* 1987; Mendlewicz *et al.* 1987).

Recombinant DNA analysis represents an entirely new way to study cancer. Somatic mutations, including translocations or deletions, sometimes together with mutations in the germline, account for some forms of both sporadic and hereditary cancers (Knudson 1986). The genes involved exist normally in cells as proto-oncogenes awaiting a stimulus to mutation to disrupt their normal regulation. Other steps may be required, and other genetic mechanisms have been suggested; cancer is not yet fully understood. Curiously, Garrod did not mention cancer in *The inborn factors in disease*. Could he have thought it an exception to chemical individuality? Whatever he thought then, today we see it as such.

All of these diseases of complex aetiology are expected to be highly heterogeneous, so it is no surprise to find genes at different loci in different families. The remarkable degree of allelic heterogeneity so well demonstrated in the LDL receptor defects is also likely to be duplicated in multifactorial disorders, so that, while groups of families may be shown to derive the genetic origin of their disease from mutations at the same locus or loci, each family may well have the distinction of their own constellations of unique mutations. Extremes of chemical individuality and genetic heterogeneity are likely to be met in families with hypertension and the psychoses, defects of especially complex homeostasis with dozens of enzymes and other proteins capable of expressing genetic variation.

As for the experience that must be involved in the transformation of latent susceptibilities into overt expression, epidemiologists are busily engaged in seeking them. But the search for risk factors is made difficult by our inability *a priori* to say risky for whom. That is, risk factors alone, whether genes or experiences, while helpful in defining potential disease in populations where they are prevalent, must be considered independently in each combination, in each individual, and in each family. A gene associated with disease in one person may not represent a real risk in another (see our example of Hartnup disorder)—and not simply because of absence of provocative experiences. Rather, since any phenotype represents the effects of all the genes entering into its origins, modifiers may nullify the potentially bad effects of any one. It will require observation of each newly discovered gene in many individuals living under many conditions before comprehensive statements of actual risks to specific individuals can be made. So the use of genetic discoveries in prevention is likely to remain a glittering prospect for some time to come. We have a long way to go on this road first proposed by Garrod.

THE CHANGING CHARACTER OF DISEASE

The human gene pool does not change significantly from one generation to the next. But the environment can and does. The major causes of disease have changed since Garrod's time because our environment is different from his.

Garrod's sons died in World War I—two in battle, one of influenza after the Armistice. The omnipresence of war generated metaphors we use in everyday language (Fussell 1975). War on disease became a concern almost equal in importance to war on a human enemy; the concern with disease began during the War between men (Fig. 4).

A metaphor is an understanding of one kind of thing in terms of another (Lakoff and Johnson 1980). Human thought processes are largely metaphorically structured and defined and metaphor means metaphorical concept. Accordingly, to use the metaphors of war in speaking of disease tells us about our concepts of disease and its causes. Garrod himself (p. 124, *Inborn factors*) used war metaphors to express his ideas:

Whilst on the one hand the *weapons of attack* have been improved by evolution, there has been a corresponding evolution of *protective mechanisms* of great ingenuity and of no small efficiency, for *the defense of the individual attacked*. [Our italics.]

Diseases and their causes are *enemies*; and *campaigns* are mounted to *conquer* them. The enemies, in the conventional view, are agents extrinsic to ourselves: 'germs and like attacking agents' and nutrient deficiencies for the large part; toxins, pollutants, and other unfriendly experiences for the remainder. The campaigns to conquer these enemies have mobilized vaccines, immunization procedures, and antibiotics; spawned concepts about minimum daily requirements for nutrients; fostered standards for cleanliness in our daily environment at work and at home. When the tactics were broadly applied to society, the incidence of diseases associated with a wide range of environmental determinants decreased. It has even been proposed in a recent book (Winter 1986) that the Great War, with its legacies of metaphors for medicine and death for human beings, reveals a paradox; the conflict which maimed and killed so many also created conditions in the civilian world which raised the standard of living and improved human health and life expectancy (Renshaw 1987).

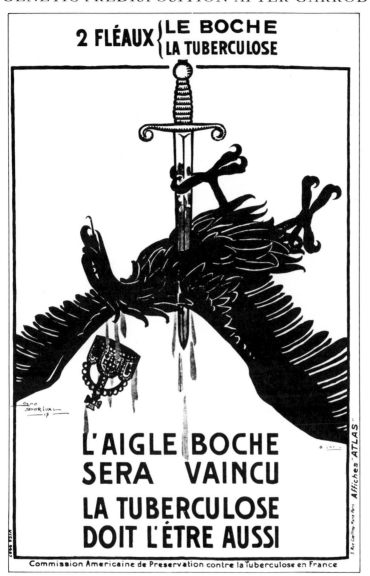

FIG. 4. A World War I poster. A visual metaphor for a concept of disease. Disease is an enemy; it can be conquered. But, if the cause of the disease is in the gene, is there an enemy? (Reproduced from Derracott 1974, p. 54.)

[211]

From this perspective, it is not surprising that the view of successful anti-disease tactics in the domain of public health has broadened into the status of a dogma. Therefore it can be very disappointing that unwanted morbidity and mortality continue despite the campaigns: too many of us are sick or die too early in life and unhealthy longevity has become a macroeconomic problem (Gori and Richter 1978). These persistent problems required an explanation and our unsatisfactory living habits filled the bill.

If disease continues in a better and cleaner environment might it be because the person is at fault—in his or her behaviour? The enemy is in a conventional locale; it remains external—in diet and inactivity and in abusive habits that bring toxins to minds and bodies. It is simply the relationship to a fair environment that is wrong. The response is to improve behaviour and abrogate cause. And to some extent, the 'lifestyle campaign' succeeds. Mortality rates decline a little further (Fig. 5). On the other hand, disease does not disappear.

When environment improves and genotype has not changed, yet disease continues, the heritability of disease has probably increased. By heritability we mean the relative importance of genetic causes among all the causes of disease in the population. We can use the case of rickets to illustrate what we mean (Scriver and Tenenhouse 1981).

Rickets is a disturbance of bone mineralization. The pathogenesis of rickets involves dishomeostasis of calcium or phosphorus metabolism. The causes of rickets are the events that undermine calcium and phosphorus homeostasis. In Garrod's lifetime, rickets was an endemic disease in the industrialized societies of temperate latitudes. Its principal cause was vitamin D deficiency related to a reduced exposure to sunlight in the winter season and insufficient sources of vitamin D in the diet in the affected person. Urbanization and atmospheric pollution accompanying smoke-stack industries were additional important 'causes' of rickets in the UK during Garrod's lifetime.

Garrod lived to know the discovery of vitamin D and the evidence that ultraviolet radiation had curative effects on rickets.

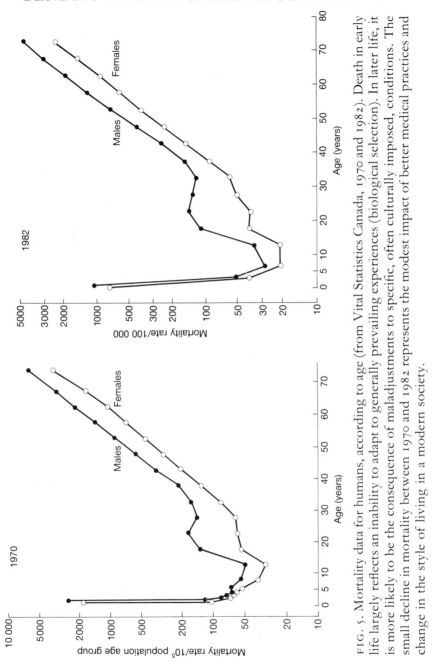

FIG. 5. Mortality data for humans, according to age (from Vital Statistics Canada, 1970 and 1982). Death in early life largely reflects an inability to adapt to generally prevailing experiences (biological selection). In later life, it is more likely to be the consequence of maladjustments to specific, often culturally imposed, conditions. The small decline in mortality between 1970 and 1982 represents the modest impact of better medical practices and change in the style of living in a modern society.

Applications of this new knowledge reduced the incidence of the disease. One year after Garrod's death, a report was published describing a patient with rickets *resistant* to vitamin D therapy (Albright *et al.* 1937). This famous report implied that rickets did not always have an external cause; it might lie in the patient's own constitution. The disease described by the Boston physicians was later shown to be a disturbance of phosphate homeostasis and its cause was mutation at a locus on the X chromosome.

The heritability of a disease increases when its major environmental causes are corrected. This was shown explicitly in the case of rickets in the population of Quebec province in Canada during the late 1960s and early 1970s. Before then, about 500 new cases were reported yearly, the majority being infants and young children. Vitamin D deficiency was the principal cause of the disease. A peculiar anomaly in the food regulations of the province prevented the practice, common elsewhere, of adding a safe supplement of vitamin D to dairy milk sold for human consumption. The aberrant Quebec regulation was changed in 1969. In the following years the incidence of rickets declined dramatically province-wide, largely because the vitamin D-deficient form of the disease was no longer overt. On the other hand, infantile rickets did not entirely disappear. A few new cases of the disease have appeared in the paediatric population every year since 1969 but their cause is different from what it was. Now they are Mendelian disorders of mineral homeostasis: about half have impaired renal synthesis of the vitamin D hormone calcitriol; the remainder have inherited renal disorders of phosphate transport. Moreover, the cases with the inborn error of vitamin D hormone biosynthesis have a 'founder effect'. The gene causing this autosomal recessive disease came to New France in a small number of families, and most current cases in Quebec are descendants of those ancestors.

This scenario satisfies medical scientists with two different points of view. Those interested in the epidemiology and incidence of disease are content that a common disease has been largely prevented; its incidence has fallen to about 2 per cent of that found before the appropriate public health measures were

[214]

taken. Those interested in genetics find that the heritability of rickets in the population has risen from a trivial value before 1969 to a high value as incidence declined. But there is a third point of view. Public health and epidemiology have little more to offer for the prevention of rickets in this population; on the other hand, knowledge about the mutations that cause rickets is now very important and necessary for the correct treatment of patients.

Rickets is a paradigm for other diseases which have both the chemical individuality and the genetic predisposition in the sense meant by Garrod. For example, phenylketonuria, congenital hypothyroidism, the fragile X syndrome, and Down syndrome are relatively more important causes of mental retardation today than they were in Garrod's lifetime. This is so because many other causes of mental retardation have been subdued by changes in medical practice: better prenatal care and higher standards of obstetrical practice to name two. The incidence of live births with these four genetic causes of mental retardation probably changed little in Garrod's lifetime and they were probably very minor causes of mental retardation in patients he would have observed in his work in paediatrics at the Hospital for Sick Children in Great Ormond Street. For Garrod and his contemporaries, they were either unrecognized entities or their cause could not be understood because the requisite knowledge was missing; 50 years later they are disorders we do not and cannot ignore.

The emphasis here is on change in the character of disease as experience changes. The relative importance of genetic contributions to disease increases as other forms of disease are controlled by the practices of public health and medicine. The search for why a particular patient has a particular disease should now lead increasingly often to an explanation in the genetic makeup of the patient. Even a disease such as acquired immune deficiency disease (AIDS), which has an unquestionable extrinsic cause (infection with the HIV-1 agent) and important components in the circumstances of infection, deserves notice from a genetic (or diathesis) point of view. Current information suggests that many have HIV infection but fewer have AIDS. Is there a reason for the few? One answer is, of course, time: the cohort of infected persons has not been followed long enough to observe appearance of the disease or the latent period may vary from one person to another. Another answer may be that some are predisposed by genotype to be relatively resistant or susceptible to infection and progression to disease. It had been proposed that polymorphism in the Gc (group specific component) blood protein is a determinant of predisposition (Eales *et al.* 1987). There are three polymorphic Gc phenotypes in man designated 1f, 1s, and 2. Among British males, it appeared only the Gc1F allele was positively associated with risk of HIV infection after exposure, progression of infection to disease, and severity of disease. No AIDS patient was Gc2 homozygous; no subject was both HIV seronegative and Gc1f homozygous after known exposure. Accordingly, perhaps Gc2 protects and Gc1f predisposed to AIDS. There has been no confirmation of these findings;* inheritance of the Gc phenotypes in AIDS patients has not been studied to rule out phenocopies, but no matter—someone is thinking about the possibility of diathesis in AIDS and that is a novel point of view on this problem, so far. Garrod would not have thought it so novel. He devoted Chapter VIII of *Inborn factors* to inherited predisposition in infective diseases.

MEDICAL EDUCATION AND MEDICAL CARE

Earlier we noted that Garrod does not mention prevention of disease in *The inborn factors*. There are good reasons why he was reticent in this regard. First, he did not know about genes or the physical basis of mutation, and, second, the lack of a clear medical goal in the contemporary eugenics movement (its goal was social) would have diverted him from seeing the merits of genetic counselling. Advances in knowledge since Garrod's lifetime have made apparent three things mentioned earlier but worth reiterating: genetic causes of disease are not rare in modern society and their expression accounts for a substantial portion of patients;

* Indeed, the finding was an artefact. But the HLA genes may influence progression of AIDS in the individual.

there are techniques to identify the causes of such disease; and there are ways to use the knowledge to avoid or prevent it.

With regard to prevalence, any estimate is suspect because there is no general agreement on what constitutes a 'genetic' disease. But with that in mind, it has been said that such diseases account for 30 per cent or more of admissions to tertiary care paediatric wards and hospitals in modern societies for example (Scriver *et al.* 1973; Hall *et al.* 1978), and an even higher proportion of admissions to some special care institutions (Gregory *et al.* 1984). Baird and colleagues (1988) used data in a vital statistics register to estimate that at least 5.3 per cent of liveborn persons can be expected to have diseases with an important genetic component before they reach 25 years of age. If multifactorial disorders occurring in the whole life-span of the population are included, the estimate is 60 per cent (UNSCEAR 1985). In addition to the 4400 Mendelian phenotypes in man, of which about three-quarters are diseases, there are several hundred recognizable congenital syndromes and malformations, the majority of which are likely to have a genetic predisposition of Mendelian or multifactorial nature. Every medical subspecialist encounters these diseases, the most likely specialists being paediatricians, neurologists, ophthalmologists, dermatologists, orthopaedic surgeons, and obstetricians (Costa *et al.* 1985). What can these physicians do about these diseases?

Garrod's physician-colleagues either could not or did not embrace his idea about genetic predisposition to disease. We can guess why this was so. The idea was either not important to them— there were other more pressing concerns; or it was not applicable—there was no way to translate the idea of genetic predisposition into a medical practice. But the circumstances have changed and they will impinge with consequences, or soon will, on every practitioner because genetics has entered the market place of medicine. Genetics did so through the development of tests and patents for procedures and materials. The tests and procedures analyse DNA composition and identify mutations and genetically linked markers of inherited predisposition to disease. This knowledge and its applications are in the public

[217]

domain and also in possession of companies who expect to profit from it. The public knows about it and any one practising medical genetics knows the public knows it, which raises several issues for physicians. First there is the large potential volume of specific tests. New tests, many still requiring validation in general practice, are described with every issue of the medical journals. Persons at risk, or who believe themselves to be at risk, will ask for the tests. Second, as long as tests are available on the market or in the health care system, their results will become available and will require interpretation. Who will interpret the tests and do the counselling? There are too few medical geneticists and genetic counsellors to meet the anticipated demand, and counselling a person about genetic predisposition takes a long time—hours not minutes in most estimates. Physicians in conventional practice don't usually have this time, and, when they do, are they able to interpret the tests and give accurate counselling? These are real problems arising from the current status of medical education and health care.

If tests indicate predispositions to disease what then is to be done? Is treatment available to prevent the disease? In most cases, the simple answer is—not yet. Will that circumstance foster more research on treatment and pathogenesis of 'genetic' disease? We hope so but we shall have to wait and see what the patrons of medical research will do. Until there is treatment, the alternative is avoidance through reproductive counselling, prenatal diagnosis, and selective pregnancy termination. The social and ethical implications in this choice, in so far as the option is available, are enormous and they preoccupy many good minds. Availability of genetic tests will also have implications for insurers and the insured, for employees and employers, wherever the purpose of the test is an issue. Physicians will be involved in all of this. Accordingly, the fact of genetic predisposition in human society has enormous implications for medical education and health care.

Medical education

Are modern physicians and other providers of health care more likely to adopt Garrod's point of view about genetic predispositions than were his colleagues? and can they? They are different questions. The answer to both is a qualified yes, if education encourages the health professional to appreciate the cogency of Garrod's great concept. Unfortunately, all the signs indicate that the curriculum does not prepare the medical graduate for Garrodian ideas revivified even though the stimuli to assimilate his ideas are everywhere apparent in medical practice.

There is little genetics in the typical medical curriculum. Surveys (Childs 1982) show that medical genetics is a minor topic in a busy curriculum; worse, it is usually treated as a categorical topic rather than as one fundamental to biology, medicine, and the understanding of human variation. Genetic thinking would have to become integral in medical thinking to assimilate Garrod's concept of chemical individuality into an awareness of genetic predisposition to disease and the typical curriculum does not encourage that trend. Disease has a rational explanation both in its pathogenesis and in its cause but the curriculum emphasizes manifestations and treatment. The scientific basis of medicine ought to attract the student's interest if it enables medicine to be rational and more science would not make medicine arid if it fostered better understanding of disease and of the patient with the disease. It has been said (Campbell 1976) that an appreciation of the nature of science and its achievements is only accidentally acquired in the traditional curriculum even though the science lead to rational treatment and prevention of disease. Familial hypercholesterolaemia, phenylketonuria, and Hartnup disorder were our examples of that point of view and genetics was their common denominator.

The genius of Garrod was in the salience of his medical thinking. It was not focused solely on diagnosis and the attendant medical activities. It was concerned with pathogenesis, limited though he was by the knowledge of his day. He perceived that a particular person had a particular disease, often under particular circumstances. In this sense Garrod's view of medicine runs utterly contrary to the conventional teaching of medicine. The latter emphasizes the disease that affects the patient; Garrod emphasized the individuality of the patient with the disease. Conventional medical teaching discourages anticipation, prevention, and avoidance of disease; Garrod's teaching encourages them.

How will medical education be changed? One might begin with human anatomy. Leonardo da Vinci saw the human body as a machine endowed with mechanical mechanisms. Vesalius followed him and through scientific enquiry laid the foundations of modern human anatomy in 1543. We have used Vesalian anatomy ever since. Now there is a neo-Vesalian anatomy, the human genome map, the micro-anatomy that is a major determinant of human form and function. Human genes, their locations on chromosomes, and their relation to each other (linkage) are becoming known and at the same time a morbid anatomy of the human genome is emerging (McKusick 1988). The repertoire of DNA tests grows steadily. Why not inculcate the medical mind with such an anatomy? Licencing and qualifying examinations that included questions on genetics might focus our minds on these aspects of medicine.

Medical care

If there is a concern that physicians are not yet prepared for roles as interpreters and counsellors, is there a corresponding concern that the health care systems of modern society can accommodate measures to deal with genetic predisposition?

Medicine is a social discipline and well-being of citizens is considered important in developed nations. Healthy citizens participate in the business of the nation. Unwell citizens exact a cost, on themselves and on the families and society to which they belong. Occurrence of disease is an uncertainty: one cannot predict which individual will have a disease and when. Garrod provided a concept that dealt with uncertainty and his concept can now be translated into practice.

The economist Kenneth S. Arrow has thought about the uncertainty of disease occurrence and the economics of medical care. He observed that medicine has a collective orientation that sets it apart from business where self-interest is the norm. Business and medical care are already in conflict in the area of genetic predisposition. It follows that government should undertake health insurance where a market fails to emerge or cannot provide what everyone needs. The failure of the market to insure against uncertainties has created many social institutions in which the usual assumptions of the market are contradicted. These observations are relevant because they bear upon the applicability of Garrod's concepts about genetic predisposition. Access to diagnostic methods, and medical thinking informed by Garrod's concepts, are required to address the issue of predisposition which is a phenomenon likely to be relevant to almost every family. Accordingly, every person may need access to the techniques of modern genetics. Unfortunately, that is not the case in health care as we know it, even though a case has been made for the cost effectiveness of molecular genetic methods in medicine (Chapple *et al.* 1987). In the American system only some, those who can afford them, can benefit from the new methods; where government health insurance operates, as in Canada, the methods are either not provided or only inadequately so. The lack of a workable universal health care system in the one society and the restricted access to expensive diagnostic methods in the other are both causes for lament (Relman 1986). How ironic that these circumstances could further delay the appearance of Garrod's ideas in medical practice.

CONCLUSION

Where will we be if and when Garrod's ideas enter the mainstream of medicine along with molecular genetic methods? One hopes that old ways of categorical thinking about disease will be gone, that the elements of heredity in disease will be recognized, and each patient will be seen as an individual with a disease. We can be certain though of the wisdom in Garrod's own cautionary note that 'in (another) 50 years a still more ample knowledge will doubtless overturn many of our own conclusions'. Let's suppose we have a complete map of the human genome in 50 years, that every gene is sequenced, its product identified, and its expression understood. What will constitute 'Still more ample knowledge' then? Genetics will have given us a detached analysis of our parts but a human being is something else. To know some or even all of our parts is not the same as to know the sum of the parts; to have the knowledge of molecular genetics and biology is one thing and to have the knowledge of physiological genetics is another. Physiological genetics is an apparent contradiction in terms: physiology is the integrative discipline concerned with homeostatic systems and genetics is the reductive discipline concerned with components of the systems and the variation in them. We need physiological genetics to understand health and its counterpart, disease. When we have it we will have come full circle to stand perhaps not in Garrod's place but at least beside him along with his contemporary Sewall Wright and the other physiological geneticists of those times.

It will become apparent that, while Beadle and others did what was obvious to them, when they reversed the thinking of their era by looking for the gene mutations that influenced known chemical reactions (and in so doing paid homage to Garrod), it will be our turn to want to know how the chemical reactions modified by mutation produce their effect on the phenotype of the whole being.

Roger Williams, a student of biological variation and admirer of Garrod, and rather like him in that he too did not see his ideas enter the mainstream of human biology, wrote this in his book *Biochemical individuality* (1958): 'The existence in every human being of a vast array of attributes which are potentially measureable (whether by present methods or not) and probably uncorrelated mathematically makes quite tenable the hypothesis that practically every human being is a deviate in some respects' (p. 3, in the 1963 Science Editions, edition). Williams saw that to understand human health is a wonderful challenge if the population, instead of being composed of individuals with normal attributes, is made up instead of individuals all of whom possess unusual attributes. The study of human individuality, he said, is an applied human biology and it could become a cornerstone of medicine with unparalleled possibilities. Garrod would surely have agreed.

BIBLIOGRAPHY OF THE WRITINGS OF ARCHIBALD E. GARROD

Based on a list (pp. 20–6) appended to an obituary notice by George Graham in *St. Bart's Hosp. Rep.*, **69**, pp. 12–19 (1936).

1882

The nebulæ: a fragment of astronomical history. Parker, Oxford, 1882. (Johnson Memorial Prize Essay of 1879; reconstructed and rewritten, 1881.)

1884

A visit to the leper hospital at Bergen (Norway). [Abstract.] *St. Bart's Hosp. Rep.*, **30**, pp. 311–13 (1884).

1885

Some cases of sclerosis of the spinal cord. *St. Bart's Hosp. Rep.*, **21**, pp. 93–9 (1885).

1886

A case of paralysis of the abductors of the vocal cords, with lesions of several cranial nerves. *St. Bart's Hosp. Rep.*, **22**, pp. 209–11 (1886).

An introduction to the use of the laryngoscope. Longmans, Green, London, 1886.

Hysteria. [Abstract.] *St. Bart's Hosp. Rep.*, **22**, p. 364 (1886).

1887

Rutpure of trachea, followed by general emphysema and asphyxia. *Med. Press. Circ.*, N.S. **45**, p. 519 (1887).

1887–8

A contribution to the theory of the nervous origin of rheumatoid arthritis. [Abstract.] *Proc. roy. med. chir. Soc. Lond.*, N.S. **2**, pp. 310–13 (1887–8).

A further contribution to the study of rheumatoid arthritis. [Abstract.] *Proc. roy. med. chir. Soc. Lond.*, N.S. **2**, pp. 372–6 (1887–8).

1888

A contribution to the theory of the nervous origin of rheumatoid arthritis. *Med.-chir. Trans.*, 2nd ser., **53**, pp. 89–105 (1888).

A further contribution to the study of rheumatoid arthritis. *Med.-chir. Trans.*, 2nd ser., **53**, pp. 265–81 (1888).

On the relation of erythema multiforme and erythema nodosum to rheumatism. *St. Bart's Hosp. Rep.*, **24**, pp. 43–54 (1888).

(Archibald E. Garrod and E. Hunt Cooke.) An attempt to determine the frequency of rheumatic family histories amongst non-rheumatic patients. *Lancet*, **ii**, p. 110 (1888).

THE WRITINGS OF ARCHIBALD E. GARROD

1889

On the relation of chorea to rheumatism, with observations of eighty cases of cholera. *Med.-chir. Trans.*, **72,** pp., 145–63 (1889).

The pathology of chorea: a suggestion. *Lancet*, **ii,** p. 1051 (1889).

1890

A treatise on rheumatism and rheumatoid arthritis, Griffin, London, 1890. Translated into French as *Traité du rhumatisme et de l'arthrite rhumatoïde. Traduit par le Dr. Brachet*, Paris [1891].

1891

A case of gouty periostitis. *Lancet*, **ii,** pp. 1334–5 (1891).

Notes on the common hæmic cardiac murmur. *St. Bart's Hosp. Rep.*, **27,** pp. 33–40 (1891).

1892

The changes in the blood in the course of rheumatic attacks. *Med.-chir. Trans.*, **75,** pp. 189–225 (1892).

On the occurrence and detection of hæmatoporphyrin in the urine. *J. Physiol.*, **13,** pp. 598–620 (1892).

On the presence of uro-hæmato-porphyrin in the urine in chorea and articulate rheumatism. *Lancet*, **i,** p. 793 (1892).

1893

On an unusual form of nodule upon the joints of the fingers. *St. Bart's Hosp. Rep.*, **29,** pp. 157–61 (1893).

On hæmatoporphyrin as a urinary pigment in disease. *J. Path. Bact.*, **1,** pp. 187–97 (1893).

1894

A contribution to the study of the yellow colouring matter of the urine. *Proc. roy. Soc.*, **55,** pp. 394–407 (1894).

On the association of cardiac malfunction with other congenital defects. *St. Bart's Hosp. Rep.*, **30,** pp. 53–61 (1894).

Some further observations on urinary hæmatoporphyrin. *J. Physiol.*, **15,** pp. 108–18 (1894).

(W. P. Herringham, A. E. Garrod, and W. J. Gow.) *A handbook of medical pathology. For the use of students in the Museum of St. Bartholomew's Hospital*, Baillière, Tindall and Cox, London, 1894.

1894–5

A contribution to the study of urœrythrin. *J. Physiol.*, **17,** pp. 439–50 (1894–5).

Hæmatoporphyrin in normal urine. *J. Physiol.*, **17,** 349–52 (1894–5).

How to look up a point in a medical library. *St. Bart's Hosp. J.*, **2,** pp. 145–6 (1894–5).

1895

Arthritis deformans. In *Twentieth century practice: an international encyclopedia of modern medical science*, Vol. 2 (ed. Stedman, Thomas L.), pp. 511–74 (1895).

THE WRITINGS OF ARCHIBALD E. GARROD

Case of a cretin under thyroid treatment. *Trans. med. Soc. Lond.*, **18**, pp. 368–9 (1895).

A case of sclerema neonatorum ending in recovery. *Lancet*, **i**, pp. 1103–5 (1895).

A case of sclerema neonatorum ending in recovery. *Trans. Med. Soc. Lond.*, **18**, pp. 314–23 (1895).

Late researches on urochrome. *Med. Press Circ.*, N.S. **59**, pp. 238–40 (1895).

The medicinal springs of Great Britain. Bath (W. M. Ord and A. E. Garrod), pp. 515–27; Buxton (W. M. Ord and A. E. Garrod), pp. 567–36; Matlock Bath, pp. 537–8; Droitwich, pp. 561–6; Nantwich, pp. 567–9; Leamington, pp. 583–8; Cheltenham, pp. 528–92; Tunbridge Wells, pp. 593–5. In *The climates and baths of Great Britain. Being the report of a committee of the Royal Medical and Chirurgical Society of London. . . .* Vol. I (1895).

A specimen of urine rendered green by indigo. *Trans. clin. Soc. Lond.*, **28**, pp. 307–9, (1895).

(A. E. Garrod and H. Morley Fletcher.) The maternal factors in the causation of rickets. *Brit. med J.*, **ii**, pp. 707–11 (1895).

(Sir Dyce Duckworth and A. E. Garrod.) A case of hepatic cirrhosis, with obstruction in the superior vena cava. *St. Bart's Hosp. Rep.*, **32**, pp. 71–7 (1895).

1896

On the pigmentation of uric acid crystals deposited from urine. *J. Path. Bact.*, **3**, pp. 100–6 (1896).

The rationale of the accepted treatment of gout. *Med. Press Circ.*, N.S. **62**, pp. 227–30 (1896).

(A. E. Garrod and F. Gowland Hopkins.) Notes on the occurrence of large quantities of hæmatoporphyrin in the urine of patients taking sulphonal. *J. Path. Bact.*, **3**, pp. 435–48 (1986); *Trans Path. Soc. Lond.*, **47**, pp. 316–34 (1896).

(A. E. Garrod and F. Gowland Hopkins.) On urobilin. Part I. The unity of urobilin. *J. Physiol.*, **20**, pp. 112–44 (1896).

[Translation.] *A treatise on cholelithiasis. By B. Naunyn. Translated by Archibald E. Garrod*, New Sydenham Society, London, 1896.

1897

A case of sclerema neonatorum. *Trans. clin. Soc. Lond.*, **30**, pp. 129–32 (1897).

Chronic rheumatism, (pp. 56–60); Muscular rheumatism, (pp. 61–4); Gonorrhœal rheumatism, (pp. 64–72); Rheumatoid arthritis [in part], (pp. 73–102). In, *A system of medicine*, Vol. 3 (ed. Allbutt, Sir Thomas Clifford), (1897).

Malformation of the aortic valves; ulcerative endocarditis; associated malformation of the liver. *Trans. path. Soc. Lond.*, **48**, pp. 42–5 (1897).

Note on the origin of the yellow pigment of urine. *J. Physiol.*, **21**, pp. 190–1 (1897).

THE WRITINGS OF ARCHIBALD E. GARROD

The spectroscopic examination of urine. *Edinb. med. J.*, N.S. **2**, pp. 105–16 (1897).

Über den Nachweis des Hämatoporphyrins im Harn. *Cbl. inn. Med.*, **18**, pp. 497–9 (1897).

(A. E. Garrod, A. A. Kanthack, and J. H. Drysdale.) On the green stools of typhoid fever, with some remarks on green stools in general. *St. Bart's Hosp. Rep.*, **33**, pp. 13–23 (1897).

[Translation.] A contribution to the clinical and bacteriological study of the Brazilian framboesia or 'boubas'. By Achilles Breda. Translated by Archibald E. Garrod. In *New Sydenham Society: Selected essays and monographs*, pp. 259–83 (1897).

[Translation.] On polypapilloma tropicum (framboesia). By M. Charlouis. Translated by Archibald E. Garrod. In *New Sydenham Society: Selected essays and monographs*, pp. 285–319 (1897).

1897–8

(F. Gowland Hopkins and A. E. Garrod.) On urobilin. Part II. The percentage composition of urobilin. *J. Physiol.*, **22**, pp. 451–64, (1897–8).

1898

Carcinoma of the œsophagus which proved fatal by perforation of the aorta. *Trans. path. Soc. Lond.*, **49**, pp. 92–3 (1898).

A case of achondroplasia. *Trans. clin. Soc. Lond.*, **31**, pp. 294–5 (1898).

1898–9

Alkaptonuria: a simple method for the extraction of homogentisinic acid from the urine. *J. Physiol.* **23**, pp. 512–14 (1898–9).

1899

A contribution to the study of alkaptonuria. *Med.-chir. Trans.*, **82**, pp. 369–94 (1899); *Proc. roy. med. chir. Soc.*, N.S. **11**, pp. 130–5 (1899).

1899–1900

Some clinical aspects of children's disease. An address delivered before the Abernethian Society, November 9th, 1899. *St. Bart's Hosp. J.*, **7**, pp. 22–5 (1899–1900).

1900

The Bradshaw Lecture on the urinary pigments in their pathological aspects. Delivered before the Royal College of Physicians of London on Nov. 6, 1900. *Lancet*, **ii**, pp. 1323–31 (1900).

(Cammidge, P. J. and A. E. Garrod.) On the excretion of diamines in cystinuria. *J. Path. Bact.*, **6**, pp. 327–33 (1900).

[Translation.] A contribution to the ætiology of tertiary syphilis, with special reference to the influence of mercurial treatment upon the development of tertiary symptoms. By Thomas v. Marchalko. Translated by Archibald

THE WRITINGS OF ARCHIBALD E. GARROD

Garrod. In *New Sydenham Society: Selected essays and monographs (from foreign sources)*, pp. 1–53 (1900).

[Translation.] Contribution to the study of visceral affections in the early stages of syphilis. I. Icterus syphiliticus precox. By O. Lasch. . . . Translated by Dr. Garrod. In *New Sydenham Society: Selected essays and monographs (from foreign sources)*, pp. 143–64 (1900).

1901

About alkaptonuria. *Lancet*, **ii,** pp. 1484–6 (1901); *Med.-Chir. Trans.*, **85,** pp. 69–77 (1902).

A case of hæmatoporphyrinuria not due to sulphonal. By James Calvert. With a report on the urine by A. E. Garrod. *Trans. clin. Soc. Lond.*, **34,** pp. 43–5 (1901).

The clinical and pathological relations of the chronic rheumatic and rheumatoid affections to acute infective rheumatism. *Lancet*, **i,** pp. 774–7 (1901).

(Sir Dyce Duckworth and A. E. Garrod.) A contribution to the study of intestinal sand, with notes on a case in which it was passed. *Med.-chir. Trans.*, **84,** pp. 389–404 (1901).

1901–2

(K. J. P. Orton and A. E. Garrod.) The benzoylation of alkapton urine. *J. Physiol.*, **27,** pp. 89–94 (1901–2).

1902

The diagnostic value of melanuria. *St. Bart's Hosp. Rep.*, **38,** pp. 25–32 (1902).

Ein Beitrag zur Kenntnis der kongenitalen Alkaptonurie. *Cbl. inn. Med.*, **23,** pp. 41–4 (1902).

The incidence of alkaptonuria: a study in chemical individuality. *Lancet*, **ii,** pp. 1616–20 (1902).

(Sir Dyce Duckworth and A. E. Garrod.) A contribution to the study of intestinal sand, with notes on a case in which it was passed. *Lancet*, **i,** pp. 653–6 (1902).

1903

The diagnostic value of melanuria. *St. Bart's Hosp. Rep.*, **38,** pp. 25–32 (1903).

Some further observations on the reaction of urochrome with acetaldehyde. *J. Physiol.*, **29,** pp. 335–40 (1903).

Ueber chemische Individualität und chemische Missbildungen. *Pflüg. Arch. ges. Physiol.*, **97,** pp. 410–18 (1903).

1903–4

Lecture introductory to a course on chemical pathology. *St. Bart's Hosp. J.*, **11,** pp. 20–2, 38–41 (1903–4).

1904

Concerning pads upon the finger joints and their clinical relationships. *Brit. med. J.*, **ii,** p. 8 (1904).

THE WRITINGS OF ARCHIBALD E. GARROD

On black urine. *Practitioner*, **72**, pp. 383–96 (1904).

A survey of the recorded cases of hæmatoporphyrinuria not due to Sulphonal. *Trans. path. Soc. Lond.*, **55**, pp. 142–51 (1904).

Tumour of the liver in a boy æt. 10 years. *Trans. clin. Soc. Lond.*, **37**, pp. 222–3 (1904).

1904–5

A clinical lecture on chorea. Delivered at the Hospital for Sick Children, Great Ormond Street, W.C. *Clin. J.*, **25**, pp. 257–63 (1904–5).

1905

Clinical diagnosis: the bacteriological, chemical, and microscopical evidences of disease. By Rudolf v. Jaksch. Fifth English edition. ... (Ed. by Archibald E. Garrod), Griffin, London, 1905.

Hæmaturia. *Trans. med. Soc. Lond.*, **28**, pp. 132–51 (1905).

(A. E. Garrod and Ll. Wynne Davies.) On a group of associated congenital malformations, including almost complete absence of the muscles of the abdominal wall, and abnormalities of the genito-urinary apparatus. *Med.-chir. Trans.*, **88**, pp. 362–81, (1905).

1905–6

(A. E. Garrod and T. Shirley Hele.) The uniformity of the homogentisic acid excretion in alkaptonuria. *J. Physiol.*, **33**, pp. 198–205 (1905–6).

(A. E. Garrod and W. H. Hurtley.) On the estimation of homogentisic acid in urine by the method of Wolkow and Baumann. *J. Physiol.*, **33**, pp. 206–10 (1905–6).

1906

Peculiar pigmetation of the skin in an infant. *Trans. clin. Soc. Lond.*, **39**, p. 216 (106).

Rheumatoid arthritis. *Practitioner*, **76**, pp. 376–87 (1906).

(A. E. Garrod and W. H. Hurtley.) Concerning cystinuria. *J. Physiol.*, **34**, pp. 217–23 (1906).

(A. E. Garrod and F. Langmead.) A case of associated congential malformations, including transposition of viscera. *Trans. clin. Soc. Lond.*, **39**, pp. 131–5 (1906).

(A. E. Garrod and F. J. Steward.) A case of primary pneumococcal peritonitis. *Lancet*, **ii**, p. 297 (1906).

1906–7

Abstract of a lecture on broncho-pneumonia in children. *St. Bart's Hosp. J.*, **14**, pp. 88–9 (1906–7).

Abstract of a lecture on chorea. *St. Bart's Hosp. J.*, **14**, pp. 88–9 (1906–7).

(A. E. Garrod and T. Shirley Hele.) A further note on the uniformity of H:N quotient in cases of alkaptonuria. *J. Physiol.*, **35**, *Proc. Physiol. Soc.*, pp. xv–xvi (1906–7).

THE WRITINGS OF ARCHIBALD E. GARROD

1907

The initial stage of myositis ossificans progressiva. *St. Bart's Hosp. Rep.*, **43,** pp. 43–9 (1907).

(A. E. Garrod and J. Wood Clarke.) A new case of alkaptonuria. *Biochem. J.*, **2,** pp. 217–20 (1907).

(A. E. Garrod and H. A. T. Fairbank.) A case of catarrhal apprendicitis due to the presence of oxyuris vermicularis. *Lancet*, **ii,** p. 772 (1907).

1907–8

A lecture on chorea. Delivered at the Hospital for Sick Children, Great Ormond Street, W.C. *Clin. J.*, **31,** pp. 1–7 (1907–8).

A lecture in empyema in children. Delivered at St. Bartholomew's Hospital. *Clin. J.*, **31,** pp. 193–7 (1907–8).

(A. E. Garrod and W. H. Hurtley.) On the supposed occurrence of uroleucic acid in the urine in some cases of alkaptonuria. *J. Physiol.*, **36,** pp. 136–41 (1907–8).

1908

Case of multiple rheumatic nodules in an adult. *Proc. roy. Soc. Med.*, **i,** i, Clin. Sect., pp. 13–14 (1908).

The Croonian lectures on inborn errors of metabolism. Delivered before the Royal College of Physicians of London on June 18th, 23rd, 25th and 30th, 1908. *Lancet*, **ii,** pp. 1–7, 73–9, 142–8, 214–20 (1908).

The initial stage of myositis ossificans progressiva. *St. Bart's Hosp. Rep.*, **43,** pp. 43–9 (1908).

(F. T. Steward and A. E. Garrod.) Case of pyo-pericardium cured by drainage. *Proc. roy. Soc. Med.*, **1,** i, Clin. Sect., pp. 15–17 (1908).

1908–9

Critical review. The excretion in the urine of sugars other than glucose. *Quart. J. Med.*, **2,** pp. 438–54 (1908–9).

Individuality in its medical aspects. Extracts from sessional address before Abernethian Society. *St. Bart's Hosp. Rep.*, **16,** pp. 18–21 (1908–9).

1909

Anomalies of urinary excretion (pp. 40–85); Uræmia (pp. 86–102). In, Osler, William, and McCrae, Thomas. *Modern medicine: its theory and practice*, Vol. 6, (1909).

Enterogenous cyanosis. In, Allbutt, Sir Clifford, and Rolleston, Humphry Davy (eds.) *A system of medicine*, Vol. 5, pp. 838–5 (1909).

Inborn errors of metabolism: the Croonian Lectures delivered before the Royal College of Physicians of London, in June, 1908. Frowde; Hodder and Stoughton, London (2nd ed.), (1909). Frowde; Hodder and Stoughton, London (1923).

Uræmia or meningitis? *Proc. roy. Soc. Med.*, **2,** i, Clin. Sect., pp. 169–75 (1909).

THE WRITINGS OF ARCHIBALD E. GARROD

1909–10

Concerning intermittent hydrarthrosis. *Quart. J. Med.*, **3**, pp. 207–20 (1909–10).

Multiple peripheral neuritis in a child. *Proc. roy. Soc. Med.*, **3**, i, Sect. Stud. Dis. Child., pp. 38–40 (1910).

1911

A case of spondylitis deformans. *Proc. roy. Soc. Med.*, **4**, i, Clin. Sect., pp. 29–30 (1911).

On auscultation of the joints. *Proc. roy Soc. Med.*, **4**, ii, Med. Sect., pp. 35–9 (1911); *Lancet*, **i**, pp. 213–14 (1911).

On the nature of the connexion between erythemata and lesions of joints. *Lancet*, **i**, pp. 1411–12 (1911).

Where chemistry and medicine meet. *Brit. med. J.*, **i**, pp. 1413–18 (1911).

1912

Lettsomian lectures on glycosuria. Delivered before the Medical Society of London. *Lancet*, **i**, pp. 483–8, 577–62, 629–35 (1912).

1912–13

The scientific spirit in medicine: inaugural sessional address to the Abernethian Society. *St. Bart's Hosp. J.*, **20**, pp. 19–27 (1912–13).

(A. E. Garrod and W. H. Hurtley.) Congenital family steatorrhœa. *Quart. J. Med.*, **6**, pp. 242–58 (1912–13).

1913

Die diätetische Behandlung der Gicht. *Med. Klin.*, **9**, pp. 1153–8 (1913).

The dietetic treatment of gout. *Lancet*, **i**, pp. 1790–4 (1913).

Discussion on non-diabetic glycosuria. Opening paper. (Eighty-first annual meeting of the British Medical Association. Held in Brighton on July 23rd, 24th, and 25th. Section of Medicine.) *Brit. Med. J.*, **ii**, pp. 850–3 (1913).

(A. E. Garrod, Frederick E. Batten, and Hugh Thursfield) (eds.) *Diseases of children, by various authors*, Arnold, London, 1913. Garrod contributed the following sections: Disease as it affects children, pp. 1–4; Diseases of the ductless glands, pp. 560–84; Disorders of metabolism, pp. 585–602. Second edition, edited by Hugh Thursfield and Donald Paterson, 1929; Garrod's section on Metabolic disorders was revised by E. A. Cockayne, pp. 530–57. Third edition, edited by Hugh Thursfield and Donald Paterson, 1934; Garrod wrote section on Inborn errors of metabolism, pp. 583–92. Fourth edition, edited by Donald Paterson and Alan Moncrieff, 2 vols., 1947–9. Fifth edition, edited by Alan Moncrieff and Philip Evans, 2 vols., 1953.

(Frew, R. S. and A. E. Garrod.) Glycosuria in tuberculous meningitis. *Lancet*, **i**, pp. 15–16 (1913).

THE WRITINGS OF ARCHIBALD E. GARROD

1914

Address in medicine delivered at the eighty-second annual meeting of the British Medical Association. *Brit. med. J.*, **ii**, pp. 228–35 (1914).

Address in medicine: on medicine from the chemical standpoint. Delivered at the eighty-second annual meeting of the British Medical Association. *Lancet*, **ii**, pp. 281–9 (1914).

Clinical applications of pathological chemistry. *Trans. internat. Cong. Med., 1913*, Sub-sect. iii (a), Chem. Path., Pt. 2, pp. 71–81 (1914).

A discussion on the thymus gland in its clinical aspects. Opening paper. (Eighty-second annual meeting of the British Medical Association. Held at Aberdeen on July 29th, 30th, and 31st. Section of Diseases of Children.) *Brit. med. J.*, **ii**, pp. 571–3 (1914).

The relations of chemistry to medicine. *Med. Press Circ.*, N.S. **98**, pp. 147–9, (1914).

(A. E. Garrod and Geoffrey Evans.) Sclerosis of the arch of the aorta, leading to obliteration of the pulses in the neck and upper limbs. *St. Bart's Hosp. Rep.*, **50**, i, pp. 65–75 (1914).

1917

A variety of war heart which calls for treatment by complete rest. *Lancet*, **i**, pp. 985–6 (1917).

1919

Islands: a lecture delivered in the Aula Magna, Malta University, 21 Jan., 1919. Malta, Empire Press, for the University, 1919.

The laboratory and the ward. *Contributions to medical and biological research dedicated to Sir William Osler in honour of his seventieth birthday July 12, 1919, by his pupils and co-workers.* New York, Vol. 1, pp. 59–69 (1919).

1919–20

A lesson in adaptation. *St. Bart's Hosp. J.*, **27**, pp. 127–8 (1919–20).

1920

On learning medicine. *Guy's Hosp. Gaz.*, **34**, pp. 336–7 (1920).

The Schorstein Lecture on the diagnosis of disease of the pancreas. Delivered at the London Hospital Medical College on February 20th, 1920. *Brit. med. J.*, **i**, pp. 459–64 (1920).

1921

Children's diseases: a retrospect. *Arch. Pediat.*, **38**, pp. 129–40 (1921).

Sir William Osler, Bart., 1849–1919. *Proc. roy. Soc.*, Series B, **92**, pp. xvii–xxiv (1921).

1921–2

(Leonard Mackey and A. E. Garrod). On congenital porphyrinuria, associated with hydroa æstivale and pink teeth. *Quart. J. Med.*, **15**, pp. 319–30 (1921–2).

[232]

THE WRITINGS OF ARCHIBALD E. GARROD

1922

A bypath of medicine (congenital porphyrinuria). *Trans. roy. med.-chir. Soc., Glasgow*, **16,** p. 165 (1922).

In memoriam. John Wickham Legg. *St. Bart's Hosp. Rep.*, **55,** pp. 1–6 (1922).

1923

Discussion on the modern treatment of diabetes. *Trans. med. Soc. Lond.*, **45,** pp. 3–4 (1923).

The Linacre Lecture entitled glimpses of the higher medicine. Delivered at Cambridge on May 5th, 1923. *Lancet*, **i,** pp. 1091–6 (1923).

1923–4

(A. E. Garrod and Geoffrey Evans.) Arthropathia psoriatica. *Quart. J. Med.*, **17,** pp. 171–8 (1923–4).

1924

The debt of science to medicine: being the Harveian Oration delivered before the Royal College of Physicians of London on St. Luke's Day 1924. Clarendon Press, Oxford, 1924.

The Harveian Oration on the debt of science to medicine. Delivered before the Royal College of Physicians of London on St. Luke's Day, October 18th. *Brit. med. J.*, **ii,** pp. 747–52 (1924).

Discussion on 'The ætiology and treatment of osteo-arthritis and rheumatoid arthritis'. *Proc. roy. Soc. Med.*, **17,** 1–11, pp. 1–4 (1924).

1924–5

Examinations from the examiner's standpoint. *St. Bart's Hosp. J.*, **32,** pp. 5–6 (1924–5).

1925

Alexander John Gaspard Marcet, Physician to Guy's Hospital, 1804–1819. *Guy's Hosp. Rep.*, **75,** pp. 373–87 (1925).

1925–6

(Leonard Mackey and A. E. Garrod.) A further contribution to the study of congenital porphyrinuria (hæmatoporphyria congenita). *Quart. J. Med.*, **19,** pp. 357–73 (1925–6).

1926

An address on the science of clinical medicine. Given at the Westminster Hospital, October 1st, 1926. *Brit. med. J.*, **ii,** pp. 621–4, (1926).

Science of clinical medicine. Delivered at the opening of the winter session of the Westminster Hospital on Oct. 1st, 1926. (Addresses to medical students. Abridged.) *Lancet*, **ii,** pp. 735–7 (1926).

1927

Congenital porphyrinuria. [Abstract.] *St. Bart's Hosp. Rep.*, **60,** p. 186 (1927).

The Huxley Lecture on diathesis. Delivered at the Charing Cross Hospital,

THE WRITINGS OF ARCHIBALD E. GARROD

November 24th, 1927. *Brit med. J.*, **ii**, pp. 967–71 (1927); *Lancet*, **ii,** pp. 1113–18 (1927).

1928

An address on the place of biochemistry in medicine. Delivered at the opening of the Courtauld Institute of Biochemistry at the Middlesex Hospital on June 14th. *Brit. med. J.*, **i**, pp. 1099–101 (1928).

The lessons of rare maladies. The Annual Oration delivered before the Medical Society of London on May 21st, 1928. *Lancet*, **i**, pp. 1055–60 (1928).

1928–9

J. F. Bullar. *(Corres.)* *St. Bart's Hosp. J.*, **36,** p. 110 (1928–9).

1929

In memoriam. Sir Dyce Duckworth, Bart., M.D., 1840–1928. *St. Bart's Hosp. Rep.*, **62,** pp. 18–30 (1929).

The power of personality. *Brit. med. J.*, **ii**, pp. 509–12 (1929).

1929–30

St. Bartholomew's fifty years ago. Summer sessional delivered to the Abernethian Society, Thursday, June 5, 1930. *St. Bart's Hosp. J.*, **37**, pp. 179–82, 200–4 (1929–30).

1931

The inborn factors in disease: an essay. Clarendon Press, Oxford, 1931.

1933–4

Chemistry and medicine. (Summary of lecture delivered to pre-clinical students.) *St. Bart's Hosp. J.*, **41,** pp. 27–8 (1933–4).

1936

Congenital porphyrinuria: a postscript. *Quart. J. Med.*, **29,** pp. 473–80 (1936).

BIBLIOGRAPHY OF ARTICLES
ABOUT A. E. GARROD

The following is a list of papers in which Garrod figures prominently. Some recount events in his life, some examine his career, others deal with his impact on modern thought.

Beadle, G. W. (1959). Genes and chemical reactions in neurospora. *Science* **129,** 1715–19.

Bearn, A. G. (1975–76). Lettsomian Lectures I. Archibald Garrod and the birth of an idea. *Medical Society Transactions* **92,** 47–56.

Bearn, A. G. (1975–76). Lettsomian Lectures II. Present concepts and future directions. *Medical Society Transactions* **92,** 57–63.

Bearn, A. G. and Miller, E. D. (1979). Archibald Garrod and the development of the concept of inborn errors of metabolism. *Bulletin of the History of Medicine* **53,** 315–28.

British Medical Journal (1936). Sir Archibald Garrod. *British Medical Journal* **1,** 731–3.

Burgio, G. R. (1986). 'Inborn errors of metabolism' and 'Chemical individuality', two ideas of Sir Archibald Garrod briefly revisited 50 years after his death. *European Journal of Pediatrics* **145,** 2–5.

Carlson, E. A. (1966). *The gene: a critical history*, pp. 66–76. Saunders, Philadelphia.

Childs, B. (1970). Sir Archibald Garrod's conception of chemical individuality: a modern appreciation. *New England Journal of Medicine* **282,** 71–7.

Childs, B. (1973). Garrod, Galton and clinical medicine. *Yale Journal of Biology and Medicine* **46,** 297–313.

Childs, B. (1985). Implications for disease of Sir Archibald Garrod's views on chemical individuality. In *Congenital metabolic diseases* (ed. R. Wapnir), pp. 3–10. M. Dekker, New York.

Childs, B., Moxon, E. R., and Winkelstein, J. A. (1989). Genetics and infectious diseases. In *The genetic basis of common disease* (ed. R. A. King, J. I. Rotter, and A. G. Motulsky). Oxford University Press, New York (in press).

Dunn, L. C. (1965). *A short history of genetics*. McGraw-Hill, New York.

Fruton, J. W. (1972). *Molecules and life*. Wiley-Interscience, New York.

Goldstein, J. L. (1986). On the origin of PAIDS (paralysed academic investigators disease syndrome). *Journal of Clinical Investigation* **78,** 848–54.

Harris, H. (1953). *An introduction to human biochemical genetics. Eugenics laboratory memoirs*, Vol. 37. Cambridge University Press, London.

[235]

THE ARTICLES ABOUT ARCHIBALD E. GARROD

Harris, H. (1963). *Garrod's Inborn errors of metabolism*. Oxford University Press, London.

Hopkins, F. G. (1936) Sir Archibald Garrod. *British Medical Journal* 1, 775–6.

Hopkins, F. G. (1936) Sir Archibald Garrod, K.C.M.G., F.R.S. *Nature* 770–1 (May 9).

Hopkins, F. G. (1938). Archibald Edward Garrod 1857–1936. *Transactions of the Royal Society* 2(6), 225–8.

Knox, W. E. (1958). Sir Archibald Garrod's 'Inborn errors of metabolism'. I. Cystinuria. *American Journal of Human Genetics* 10, 3–32.

Knox, W. E. (1958). Sir Archibald Garrod's 'Inborn errors of metabolism'. II. Alkaptonuria. *American Journal of Human Genetics* 10, 95–124.

Knox, W. E. (1958). Sir Archibald Garrod's 'Inborn errors of metabolism'. IV. Pentosuria. *American Journal of Human Genetics* 10, 385–97.

Knox, W. E. (1967). Sir Archibald Garrod. *Genetics* 56, 1–6.

Lancet (1936). Sir Archibald Edward Garrod, K.C.M.G., M.D., F.R.S., *Lancet* i, 807–9.

Needham, J. and Baldwin, E. (Eds.) (1949) *Hopkins and biochemistry 1861–1947*. Cambridge, UK.

Olby, R. (1974). *The path to the double helix*, pp. 123–43. University of Washington Press, Seattle.

Penrose, L. S. (1950). Garrod's conception of inborn error and its development. *Biochemical Society Symposium*, No. 4, p. 10. Cambridge University Press, Cambridge.

Peters, R. A. (1958). Some reminiscences of Sir Archibald Garrod, K.C., F.R.C.P., F.R.S. *American Journal of Human Genetics* 10, 1–2.

Scriver, C. R. (1976). Genetics: voyage of discovery for everyman. *Pediatric Research* 10, 865–72.

Scriver, C. R. (1985). Inborn errors of metabolic homeostasis: Garrod's message revisited. In *Congenital metabolic disease* (ed. R. Wapnir), pp. 11–40. M. Dekker, New York.

Sinohara, H. (1980). Archibald Garrod: a biographical essay. *Seikagaku* 52, 1155–72.

St. Bartholomew's Hospital Reports (1936). Sir Archibald E. Garrod, K.C.M.G., D.M., F.R.C.P., F.R.S., 1858–1936. *St. Bartholomew's Hospital Reports* 69, 12–16.

Vella, F. (1965). Sir Archibald Garrod's stay in Malta 1915–1919. *St. Bartholomew's Hospital Journal* (April) 1–8.

Vella, F. (1968). Sir Archibald Garrod and Malta. A historical occasion recalled. *St. Luke's Hospital Gazette* 1, 41–50.

Vella, F. (1968). 'The university of Utopia'. A lecture given by Sir Archibald Garrod, 3rd November 1917, Malta. *St. Luke's Hospital Gazette* 4, 122–7.

REFERENCES

Albright, F., Butler, A. H., and Bloomberg, G. (1937). Rickets resistant to vitamin D therapy. *American Journal of Diseases of Children* **59,** 529–47.

Allbutt, C. and Rolleston, H. D. (1910). *A system of Medicine.* Macmillan, London.

Baird, P. A., Anderson, T. W., Newcombe, H. B., and Lowry, R. B. Genetic disorders in children and young adults. A population study. (1988). *American Journal of Human Genetics* **42,** 677–93.

Baron, D. N., Dent, C. E., Harris, H., Hart, E. W., and Jepson, J. B. (1956). Hereditary pellagra-like skin rash with temporary cerebellar ataxia, constant renal aminoaciduria and other bizarre biochemical features. *Lancet* ii, 421–8.

Bateson, W. (1926). Segregation. Joseph Leidy Lecture. *American Naturalist* **16,** 201–35.

Bateson, W. (1901–02). *Report of the Evolution Committee of the Royal Society* **1,** 133.

Beadle, G. W. (1945). Biochemical genetics. *Chemical Reviews* **37,** 15–96.

Beadle, G. W. (1959). Genes and chemical reactions in Neurospora. *Science* **129,** 1715–19.

Bearn, A. G. and Miller, E. D. (1979). Archibald Garrod and the development of the concept of inborn errors of metabolism. *Bulletin of the History of Medicine* **53,** 315–28.

Biozzi, G., Mouton, D., Stiffel, C., and Bouthillier, Y. (1984). Major role of macrophases in quantitative genetic regulation of immuno-responsiveness and anti-infections immunity. *Advances in Immunology* **36,** 189–234.

Brady, R. O. and Barranger, J. A. (1983). Glucosylceramide lipidosis: Gaucher's disease. In *The metabolic basis of inherited disease,* 5th edn. (ed. J. B. Stanbury, J. B. Wyngaarden, D. S. Fredrickson, J. L. Goldstein, and M. S. Brown), pp. 831–41. McGraw-Hill, New York.

British Medical Journal (1932a). Biochemistry in medicine. *British Medical Journal* **1,** 524–5.

British Medical Journal (1932b). The struggle for health. *British Medical Journal* **1,** 713–14.

British Medical Journal (1936). Sir Archibald Garrod. *British Medical Journal* **1,** 731–3.

Brown, M. S. and Goldstein, J. L. (1986). A receptor-mediated pathway for cholesterol homeostasis. *Science* **232,** 34–47.

Byers, P. H. and Bonadio, J. F. (1985). The molecular basis of clinical heterogeneity in osteogenesis imperfecta. In *Genetic and metabolic disease in pediatrics* (ed. J. K. Lloyd and C. R. Scriver), pp. 59–90. Butterworths, London.

REFERENCES

Campbell, E. J. M. (1976). Basic science, science and medical education. *Lancet* **i**, 134–6.

Cannon, W. B. (1932). *The wisdom of the body*. W. W. Norton, New York.

Chapple, J. C., Dale, R., and Evans, B. G. (1987). The new genetics: will it pay its way? *Lancet* **i**, 1189–92.

Childs, B. (1982). Genetics in the medical curriculum. *American Journal of Medical Genetics* **13**, 319–24.

Childs, B. (1983). Causes of essential hypertension. *Progress in Medical Genetics* **5** (New Series), 1–34.

Childs, B., Moxon, E. R., and Winkelstein, J. A. (1989). Genetics and infectious diseases. In *The genetics of common diseases* (ed. R. A. King, J. I. Rotten, and A. G. Motulsky). Oxford University Press, New York (in press).

Costa, T., Scriver, C. R., and Childs, B. (1985). The effect of Mendelian disease on human health: a measurement. *American Journal of Medical Genetics* **21**, 231–42.

Deeb, S., Failos, A., Brown, B. G., Brunzell, J. D., Albers, J. J., and Motulsky, A. G. (1986). Molecular genetics of apolipoproteins and coronary heart disease. *Cold Spring Harbor Symposium, Quart. Biol.* **51**, 403–9.

Denniston, C. (1982). Low level radiation and genetic risk estimates in man. *Annual Review of Genetics* **16**, 329–55.

Dent, C. E., and Rose, G. A. (1951). Amino acid metabolism in cystinuria. *Quarterly Journal of Medicine* **79**, 205–20.

Derracott, J. (1974). *The First World War in posters*. Dover Publications, New York.

DiLella, A. G. and Woo, S. L. C. (1987). Molecular basis of phenylketonuria and its clinical applications. *Molecular Biology and Medicine* **4**, 183–92.

Eales, L.-J., Nye, K. E., Parkin, J. H., Weber, J. N., Forster, S. M., Harris, J. R. W., and Pinching, A. J. (1987). Association of different allelic forms of group specific component with susceptibility to and clinical manifestation of human immunodeficiency virus infection. *Lancet* **i**, 999–1002.

Egeland, J. A., Gearhart, D. S., Pauls, D. L., Sussex, J. N., Kidd, K. K., Allen, C. R., Hostetter, A. M., and Housman, D. E. (1987). Bipolar affective disorders linked to DNA markers on chromosome 11. *Nature* **325**, 783–7.

Fölling, A. (1934). Über Ausscheidung von Phenylbrenztraubensaüre in den Harn als Stoffwechselanomalie in Verbindung mit Imbezillität. *Zeitschrift für Physiologie und Chemische* **227**, 169–76.

Froggatt, P. and Nevin, N. C. (1971). The 'Law of Ancestral Heredity' and the Mendelian-ancestrian controversy in England, 1899–1906. *Journal of Medical Genetics* **8**, 1–36.

Fruton, J. S. (1972). *Molecules and life*, pp. 148–79, 225–61. Wiley-Interscience, New York.

REFERENCES

Fussel, P. (1975). *The Great War and modern memory*. Oxford University Press, London.

Garrod, A. E. (1902). The incidence of alkaptonuria. A study in chemical individuality. *Lancet* **ii**, 1616–20.

Garrod, A. E. (1908). The Croonian lectures on inborn errors of metabolism. *Lancet* **ii**, I, (Albinism) pp. 1–7; II, (Alkaptonuria) pp. 73–9; III, (Cystinuria) pp. 142–8; IV, (Pertosuria) pp. 214–20.

Garrod, A. E. (1909). *Inborn errors of metabolism*. Henry Frowde, Hodder and Stoughton, London. (Second edition 1923.)

Goldbourt, V. and Neufeld, H. N. (1986). Genetic aspects of arteriosclerosis. *Arteriosclerosis* **6**, 357–77.

Goldstein, J. L. (1986). On the origins of PAIDS (paralyzed academic investigator's disease syndrome). *Journal of Clinical Investigation* **78**, 848–54.

Goldstein, J. L., Hazzard, W. R., Schrott, H. G., Bierman, E. L., Motulsky, A. G., Levinski, M. J., and Campbell, E. D. (1973*a*). Hyperlipidemia in coronary heart disease. I. Lipid levels in 500 survivors of myocardial infarction. *Journal of Clinical Investigation* **52**, 1533–43.

Goldstein, J. L., Schrott, H. G., Hazzard, W. R., Bierman, E. L., Motulsky, A. G., Campbell, E. D., and Levinski, M. J. (1973*b*). Hyperlipidemia in coronary heart disease. II. Genetic analysis of lipid levels in 176 families and delineation of a new inherited disorder, combine hyperlipidemia. *Journal of Clinical Investigation* **52**, 1544–68.

Gori, G. B. and Richter, B. J. (1978). Macroeconomics of disease. Prevention in the United States. *Science* **200**, 1124–30.

Gregory, D., Kaplan, P., and Scriver, C. R. (1984). Genetic causes of chronic musculoskeletal disease in children are common. *American Journal of Medical Genetics* **19**, 533–8.

Haldane, J. B. S. (1937). The biochemistry of the individual. In *Perspectives in biochemistry* (ed. J. Needham and D. E. Green), pp. 1–10. Cambridge University Press, Cambridge.

Hall, J. G., Powers, E. K., McIlvaine, R. T., and Ean, V. H. (1978). The frequency of financial burden of genetic disease in a pediatric hospital. *American Journal of Medical Genetics* **1**, 417–36.

Harris, H. (1963). *Garrod's inborn errors of metabolism*. Oxford University Press, London.

Harris, H. (1980). *The principles of human biochemical genetics*, 3rd edn., pp. 316–405. Elsevier, London.

Harris, H., Mittwoch, U., Robson, E. B., and Warren, F. L. (1955). Phenotypes and genotypes in cystinuria. *Annals of Human Genetics* **20**, 57–91.

Harvey, H. M. (1986). *The Association of American Physicians, 1886–1986. A century of progress in medicine*. Johns Hopkins University Press, Baltimore, Maryland.

Hobbs, H. H., Brown, M. S., Russell, D. W., Davignon, J., and Goldstein,

REFERENCES

J. L. (1987). Deletion in the gene for the low-density-lipoprotein receptor in a majority of French Canadians with familial hypercholesterolemia. *New England Journal of Medicine*, **317**, 734–7.

Hopkins, F. G. (1936*a*). Sir Archibald Garrod. *British Medical Journal* **1**, 775–6.

Hopkins, F. G. (1936*b*). Sir Archibald Garrod, K.C.M.G., F.R.S. *Nature* 770–1 (May 9).

Hopkins, F. G. (1938). Archibald Edward Garrod 1857–1936. *Transactions of the Royal Society* **2**(6), 225–8.

Jeffreys, A. J., Wilson, V., and Thein, S. L. (1985). Individual-specific fingerprints of human DNA. *Nature* **316**, 76–9.

Jepson, J. B. (1978). Hartnup disease. In *The metabolic basis of inherited disease* 5th edn. (ed. J. B. Stanbury, J. B. Wyngaarden, D. S. Fredrickson, J. L. Goldstein, and M. S. Brown), pp. 1563–77. McGraw-Hill, New York.

Journal of the American Medical Association (1931). The inborn factors in disease. *Journal of the American Medical Association* **97**, 1174.

King, L. S. (1982). *Medical thinking. A historical preface*, pp. 175–7. Princeton University Press, Princeton, New Jersey.

Knudson, A. G., Jr (1986). Genetics of human cancer. *Annual Reviews of Genetics* **20**, 231–51.

Lakoff, G. and Johnson, M. (1980). *Metaphors we live by*, pp. 3–6. University of Chicago Press, Chicago.

Lancet (1932). The inborn factors in disease. *Lancet* **i**, 939.

Lancet (1936). Sir Archibald Edward Garrod, K.C.M.G., M.D., F.R.S. *Lancet* **i**, 807–9.

Lander, E. R. and Botstein, D. (1987). Homozygosity mapping: a way to map human recessive traits with the DNA of inbred children. *Science* **236**, 1567–70.

Lewontin, R. C. (1985). Population genetics. *Annual Review of Genetics* **19**, 81–102.

Lux, S. E. (1983). Disorders of the red cell membrane skeleton: hereditary spherocytosis and hereditary elliptocytosis. In *The metabolic basis of inherited disease*, 5th edn. (ed. J. B. Stanbury, J. B. Wyngaarden, D. S. Fredrickson, J. L. Goldstein and M. S. Brown), pp. 1573–605. McGraw-Hill, New York.

Matsunaga, F. (1982). Perspectives in mutation epidemiology. I. Incidence and prevalence of genetic disease (excluding chromosomal aberrations) in human populations. *Mutation Research* **99**, 95–128.

Mayr, E. (1961). Cause and effect in biology. *Science* **134**, 1501–6.

Mayr, E. (1980). Some thoughts on the history of the evolutionary synthesis. In *The evolutionary synthesis* (ed. E. Mayr and W. Provine)., pp. 1–48. Harvard University Press, Cambridge, Massachusetts.

McCrae, T. (Ed.) (1935). *Osler's principles and practice of medicine*, 12th edn. Appleton-Century, New York.

[240]

REFERENCES

McDevitt, H. O. (1985). The HLA system and its relation to disease. *Hospital Practice*, 57–72 (July 15).

McKusick, V. A. (1983). *Mendelian inheritance in man. Catalogs of autosomal dominant, autosomal recessive, and X-linked phenotypes*, 6th edn., Appendix I, Part B. Johns Hopkins Press, Baltimore, Maryland.

McKusick, V. A. (1988). *Mendelian inheritance in man. Catalogs of autosomal dominant, autosomal recessive, and X-linked phenotypes*, 8th edn., pp. lxxx–lxxxi. Johns Hopkins University Press, Baltimore, Maryland.

Medes, G. (1932). A new error of tyrosine metabolism: tyrosinosis. The intermediary metabolism of tyrosine and phenylalanine. *Biochem. J.* **26**, 917–40.

Meindl, R. S. (1982). Components of longevity: developmental and genetic responses to differential childhood mortality. *Social Science and Medicine* **16**, 165–74.

Mendlewicz, J., Simon, P., Sevy, S., Charon, F., Brocas, H., Legros, S., and Vassart, G. (1987). Polymorphic DNA marker on X chromosome and manic depression. *Lancet* **i**, 1230–2.

Merton, R. K. (1961). Singletons and multiples in scientific discovery. *Proceedings of the American Philosophical Society* **102**, 470–86.

Monk, M. (1987). Memories of mother and father. *Nature* **328**, 203–4.

Moore, J. A. (1986). Science as a way of knowing. III. Genetics. *American Zoologist* **26**, 583–747.

Motulsky, A. G. (1957). Drug reactions, enzymes and biochemical genetics. *Journal of the American Medical Association* **165**, 835–7.

Muller, H. J. (1927). Artificial transmutation of the gene. *Science* **66**, 84–7.

Murphy, E. A. and Pyeritz, R. E. (1986). Homeostasis VII. A conspectus. *American Journal of Medical Genetics* **24**, 735–51.

Needham, J. (1962). Frederick Gowland Hopkins. *Perspectives in Biology and Medicine* **6**, 2–46.

New England Journal of Medicine (1932). The inborn factors in disease. *New England Journal of Medicine* **206**, 1016.

Olby, R. (1974). *The path to the double helix*, pp. 123–43, 435. University of Washington Press, Seattle.

Osler, W. and McCrae, T. (1925). *Modern medicine*, 3rd edn. Lea and Febiger, London.

Petersdorf, R. G., Adams, R. D., Braunwald, E., Isselbacher, K. J., Martin, J. B., and Wilson, J. D. (Eds.) (1983). *Harrison's principles of internal medicine*, 10th edn. McGraw-Hill, New York.

Petersen, G. M., Silimperi, D. R., Scott, E. M., Hall, D. B., Rotter, J. I., and Ward, J. I. (1985). Uridine monophosphate kinase 3: a genetic marker for susceptibility to hemophilus influenzae type B disease. *Lancet* **ii**, 417–18.

Reeders, S. T., Breuning, M. H., Davies, K. E., Nicholls, R. D., Jarman,

REFERENCES

A. P., Higgs, D. R., Pearson, P. L., and Weatherall, D. J. (1985). A highly polymorphic DNA marker linked to adult polycystic kidney disease on chromosome 16. *Nature* **317**, 542–4.

Relman, A. S. (1986). The United States and Canada: Different approaches to health care. *New England Journal of Medicine* **315**, 1608–10.

Renshaw, P. (1987). *The Times Literary Supplement* May 15, 1987, p. 510.

Rolleston, H. D. (1927). *Idiosyncracies*. Kegan Paul, London.

Rose, G. (1985). Sick individuals and sick populations. *International Journal of Epidemiology* **14**, 32–8.

Ryder, L. P., Svejgaard, A., and Dausset, J. (1981). Genetics of HLA disease association. *Annual Review of Genetics* **15**, 169–88.

Scott-Moncrieff, R. (1981–83). The classical period in chemical genetics. *Notes and Records of the Royal Society of London* **36–7**, 125–54.

Scriver, C. R. and Clow, C. L. (1980). Phenylketonuria: epitome of human biochemical genetics. *New England Journal of Medicine* **303**, 1336–42, 1394–400.

Scriver, C. R., and Tenenhouse, H. S. (1981). On the heritability of rickets, a common disease (Mendel, mammals and phosphate). *The Johns Hopkins Medical Journal* **149**, 179–87.

Scriver, C. R., Neal, J. L., Saginur, R., and Clow, A. (1973). The frequency of genetic disease and congenital malformation among patients in a pediatric hospital. *Canadian Medical Association Journal* **108**, 1111–15.

Scriver, C. R., Mahon, B., Levy, H. L., Clow, C. L., Reade, T. M., Kronick, J., Lemieux, B., and Laberge, C. (1987). The Hartnup phenotype: Mendelian transport disorder, multifactorial disease. *American Journal of Human Genetics* **40**, 410–12.

Sly, W. S., Whyte, M. P., Sundaram, V., Tashian, R. E., Hewett-Emmett, D., Guibaud, P., Vainsel, M., Baluarte, H. J., Gruskin, A., Al-Mosawi, M., Sakati, N., and Ohlsson, A. (1985). Carbonic anhydrase II deficiency in 12 families with the autosomal recessive syndrome of osteopetrosis with renal tubular acidosis and cerebral calcification. *New England Journal of Medicine* **313**, 139–45.

Sober, E. (1984). *The nature of selection. Evolutionary theory in philosophical focus*, pp. 87–102. MIT Press, Cambridge MA.

St. George-Hyslop, P., Tanzi, R. E., Polinsky, R. J., Haines, J. L., Nee, L., Watkins, P. C., Myers, R. H., Feldman, R. G., Pollen, D., Drachman, D., Growdon, J., Bruni, A., Foncin, J-F., Salmon, D., Frommelt, P., Amaducci, L., Sorbi, S., Piacentini, S., Stewart, G. D., Hobbs, W. J., Conneally, P. M., and Gusella, J. F. (1987). The genetic defect causing familial Alzheimer's disease maps on chromosome 21. *Science* **235**, 885–9.

Stanbury, J. B., Wyngaarden, J. B., Fredrickson, D. S., Goldstein, J. L., and Brown, M. S. (Eds.) (1983). *The metabolic basis of inherited disease*, 5th edn. McGraw-Hill, New York.

REFERENCES

Stent, G. S. (1972). Prematurity and uniqueness in scientific discovery. *Scientific American* **227**, 84–93.

Tanzi, R. E., Gusella, J. F., Watkins, P. C., Bruns, G. A. P., St George-Hyslop, P., Van Keuren, M. L., Patterson, D., Pagen, S., Kurnit, D. M., and Neve, R. L. (1987). Amyloid B protein gene: cDNA, mRNA distribution, and genetic linkage near the Alzheimer locus. *Science* **235**, 880–4.

Temkin, O. (1963). The scientific approach to disease: specific entity and individual sickness. In *Scientific change* (ed. A. C. Crombie), pp. 629–47. Basic Books, New York.

Trevor-Roper, P. D. (1952). Marriage of two complete albinos with normally pigmented offspring. *British Journal of Ophthalmology* **36**, 107.

Troland, L. T. (1917). Biological enigmas and the theory of enzyme action. *American Naturalist* **51**, 321–50.

UNSCEAR Report (1985). *Genetic and somatic effects of ionizing radiation*. United Nations, New York.

Vogel, F. (1959). Moderne Probleme der Humangenetik. *Ergebnisse Innere Medizinisohe Kinderheilkunde* **12**, 52–125.

Watkins, J. F. (1986). *The Times Literary Supplement*. Sept. 19, 1986, p. 1024.

Williams, R. J. (1956). *Biochemical individuality. The basis for the genetotrophic concept*. John Wiley and Sons, New York. (Science Editions, 1963, p. 3.)

Winter, J. M. *The Great War and the British people*. London. Macmillan. 1986.

Wright, S. (1917). Color inheritance in mammals. *Journal of Heredity* **8**, 224–35.

Wright, S. (1941). The physiology of the gene. *Physiological Reviews* **21**, 487–527.

Ziman, J. (1979). *Reliable knowledge. An explanation of the grounds for belief in science*. Cambridge University Press, New York.

INDEX

INDEX

INDEX

hydroquinone-acetic acid 137
hyperchlorhydria 105
hypercholesterolaemia, *see* familial
    hypercholesterolaemia
hypersensitivity 58–9, 158–60
    see also allergies; anaphylaxis
hypertension 207
hyperthyroidism 59
hypothyroidism 59

ichthyosis 107
idiosyncrasies 156–69
    Rolleston definition 157
immunity 54
immunity, relative natural 44
The inborn factors in disease
    a facsimile of 25–184
    original index to 182–4
    reactions to 20–2
individuality 48
    and PKU 200
infection 54, 81–3, 146–56
    definition of 148
    see also bacteria
influenza 152

jaundice 90, 112, 119

kerasin 114
kidney 71, 80, 102

laboratory methods 47
Lamarck theory 77
larynx papilloma 95
LDL receptors 194–6, 209
lead 52, 87
lecithins 19, 65
leprosy 39
leucine 127
leukaemia 39
Liebig 9
lovostatin 194
lymphatic leukaemia 95
lysine 127

malformation 101–3
manic-depressive disorder 208
measles 82, 174
Meckel's diverticulum 103–4
medical care 220–1
medical education 216–19
medicine 12–16

Mendelian theory 3, 5, 10–11, 18, 68, 85,
    87–8, 90, 110, 114, 131, 137, 142, 154,
    173, 207
melanin 144
meningitis 51
mercapturic acid 81, 149
metabolic disease 120–46
mevinolin 194
MHC 207
molecules 65–6
'Mongolian idiocy' 94
'morbid liabilities', inheritance of 84–97
Morgan School of Genetics 10
"Multiplier" (Merton, history) 18, 19
muscular dystrophy 60, 90, 177
mutations 7, 16, 65–6, 73, 84, 172
myatonia congenita 95
myositis ossificans 110–11
myxoedema 41, 59, 174

nervous system disease 60
neuro-muscular abiotrophies 115–18
nominalist concept of disease 16
nucleotides 19

obesity 39
oechronosis 138, 143–4
ontological concept of disease 16
Osler, Sir William 4
osteoarthritis 110, 135–6
osteosclerosis 109
oxaluria 39

pancreatic cancer 60
pentosuria 178
pernicious anaemia 100
phenylalanine 80, 137
    and PKU 197–201
phenylketonuria (PKU) 13, 197–201
phenylpyruvic oligophrenia, *see*
    phenylketonuria (PKU)
phosphaturia 39
pigmentation 18, 88–90, 139–44
PKU, *see* phenylketonuria
pneumococcal infections 56, 61
pneumonia 48, 56, 61, 92, 95
poliomyelitis 61
porphyria 177
porphyrins 119, 141–2
porphyrinuria 7, 13, 142–3
precipitin test 67
'precursor disease' (Olby, history) 17
'predestination' to disease 97

INDEX